Surgical Care

made

Incredibly Visual!™

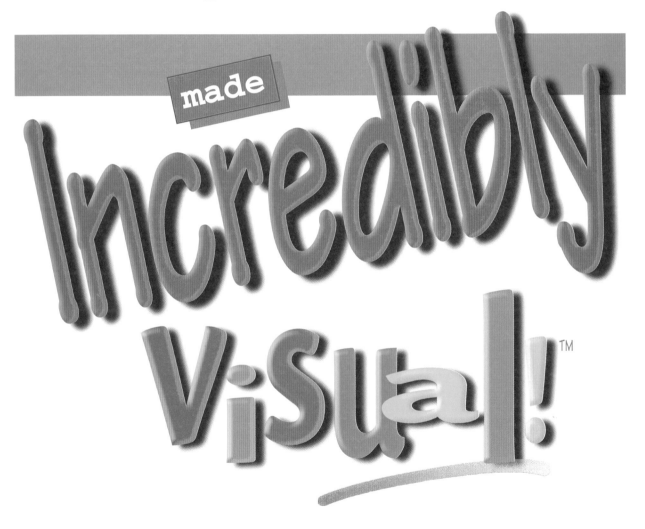

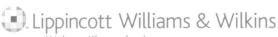
Lippincott Williams & Wilkins
a Wolters Kluwer business

Philadelphia · Baltimore · New York · London
Buenos Aires · Hong Kong · Sydney · Tokyo

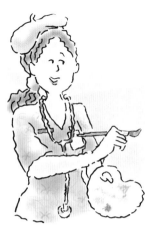

Staff

Executive Publisher
Judith A. Schilling McCann, RN, MSN

Editorial Director
David Moreau

Clinical Director
Joan M. Robinson, RN, MSN

Senior Art Director
Arlene Putterman

Art Director
Mary Ludwicki

Senior Managing Editor
Jaime Stockslager Buss, ELS

Clinical Manager
Collette Bishop Hendler, RN, BS, CCRN

Editorial Project Manager
Coleen M.F. Stern

Clinical Project Manager
Mary Perrong, RN, CRNP, MSN, APRN,BC

Editor
Kathy Goldberg

Copy Editors
Kimberly Bilotta (supervisor), Shana Harrington,
Dorothy P. Terry, Pamela Wingrod

Designer
Lynn Foulk

Illustrators
Joseph John Clark, Jacqueline Facciolo,
Judy Newhouse, Leah Rhoades Purvis,
Betty Winnberg

Digital Composition Services
Diane Paluba (manager), Joyce Rossi Biletz

Associate Manufacturing Manager
Beth J. Welsh

Editorial Assistants
Megan L. Aldinger, Karen J. Kirk, Linda K. Ruhf

Design Assistants
Georg W. Purvis, IV; Eoanna Larsen

Indexer
Karen C. Comerford

The clinical treatments described and recommended in this publication are based on research and consultation with nursing, medical, and legal authorities. To the best of our knowledge, these procedures reflect currently accepted practice. Nevertheless, they can't be considered absolute and universal recommendations. For individual applications, all recommendations must be considered in light of the patient's clinical condition and, before administration of new or infrequently used drugs, in light of the latest package-insert information. The authors and publisher disclaim any responsibility for any adverse effects resulting from the suggested procedures, from any undetected errors, or from the reader's misunderstanding of the text.

The publishers have made every effort to obtain permission from the copyright holders to use borrowed material. If any material requiring permission has been overlooked, the publishers will be pleased to make the necessary arrangements at the first opportunity.

SCIV010606—061211

Library of Congress Cataloging-in-Publication Data

Surgical care made incredibly visual.
    p. ; cm.
    Includes bibliographical references and index.
1. Therapeutics, Surgical — Atlases. 2. Therapeutics, Surgical — Handbooks, manuals, etc. 3.Surgical nursing — Atlases. 4. Surgical nursing — Handbooks, manuals, etc. I. Lippincott Williams & Wilkins.
[DNLM: 1. Perioperative Care — methods — Atlases. 2. Perioperative Care — methods — Handbooks. 3. Preoperative Care — methods — Atlases. 4. Preoperative Care — methods — Handbooks. WO 39 S95978 2007]
RD49.S866 2007
617'.919 — dc22
ISBN13 978-1-58255-946-9
ISBN10 1-58255-946-5 (alk. paper)   2006004709

Contents

On Broadway   iv

Contributors and consultants   vi

1   **Preoperative care**   1

2   **Fundamentals of anesthesia**   19

3   **Perioperative care**   39

4   **Procedures**   63

5   **Perianesthesia care**   123

6   **Postoperative care**   147

Selected references   195

Credits   197

Index   198

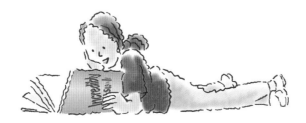

ON BROADWAY

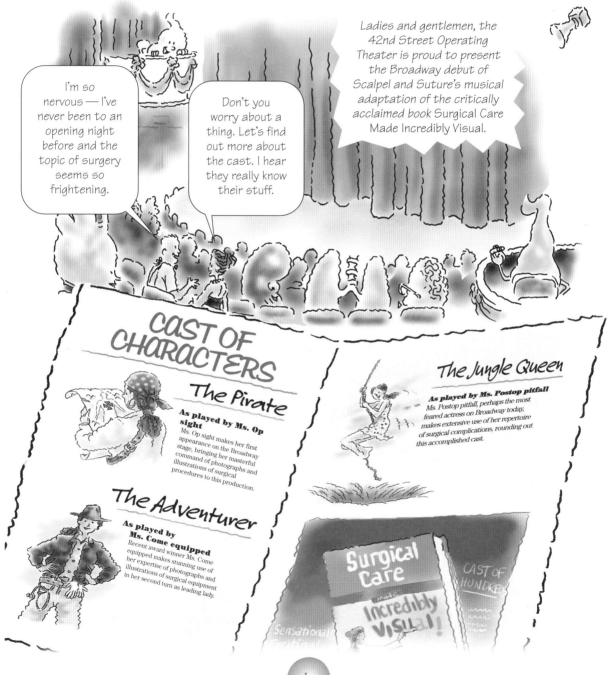

I'm so nervous — I've never been to an opening night before and the topic of surgery seems so frightening.

Don't you worry about a thing. Let's find out more about the cast. I hear they really know their stuff.

Ladies and gentlemen, the 42nd Street Operating Theater is proud to present the Broadway debut of Scalpel and Suture's musical adaptation of the critically acclaimed book Surgical Care Made Incredibly Visual.

CAST OF CHARACTERS

The Pirate

As played by Ms. Op sight
Ms. Op sight makes her first appearance on the Broadway stage, bringing her masterful command of photographs and illustrations of surgical procedures to this production.

The Adventurer

As played by Ms. Come equipped
Recent award winner Ms. Come equipped makes stunning use of her expertise of photographs and illustrations of surgical equipment in her second turn as leading lady.

The Jungle Queen

As played by Ms. Postop pitfall
Ms. Postop pitfall, perhaps the most feared actress on Broadway today, makes extensive use of her repertoire of surgical complications, rounding out this accomplished cast.

Surgical Care

Incredibly VISUAL!

Sensational

CAST OF HUNDKED

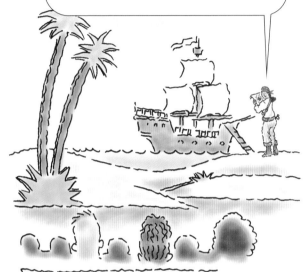

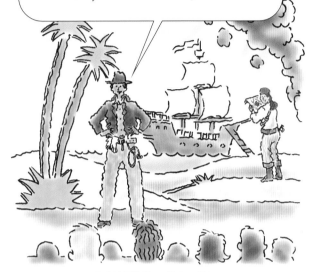

...hours later

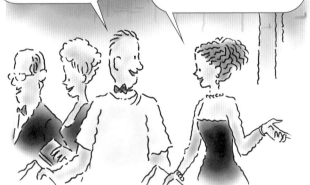

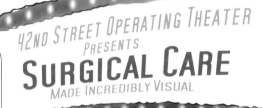

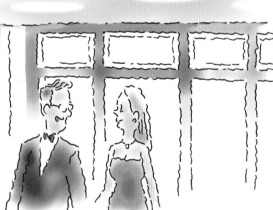

Contributors and consultants

Mary-Rita Blute, RN, MS, CPAN
Research Nurse/Program Coordinator II
Department of Anesthesiology & Critical
  Care Medicine
School of Medicine
Johns Hopkins University
Baltimore

Tina Clontz, RN, CPAN
Staff Nurse
Orlando (Fla.) Regional Medical Center

Lakshmi McRae, RN, C, BA (H)
Staff Nurse
Shriner's Hospital for Children,
  Galveston (Tex.)

Susan D. Sheets, RN, BSN, CNOR
Program Chair Surgical Technology
Ivy Tech Community College of Indiana
Columbus

Paulette C. Watts, RN, BSN, CNOR, LMT
Nurse Administrator
Summit Surgery Center
Covington, La.

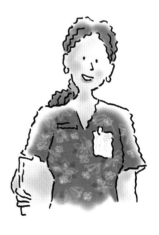

1

Preoperative care

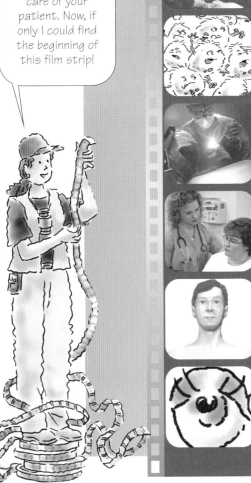

We begin with the preoperative care of your patient. Now, if only I could find the beginning of this film strip!

History of surgery 2

Surgical team 4

Informed consent 5

Phases of surgery 6

Diagnostic testing 7

Preoperative assessment 8

Anesthesia evaluation 12

Patient teaching 14

Preoperative verification 16

Vision quest 18

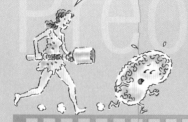

> I know this trephine looks scary, but it should ease your headache.

History of surgery

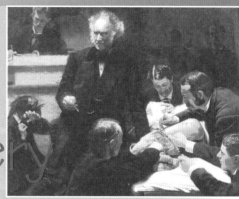

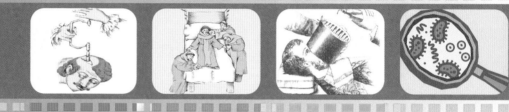

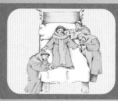

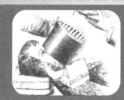

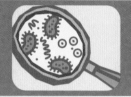

Prehistoric times

Cave drawings dating back to 3500 B.C. show trephining of the skull, the first known surgical procedure.

The trephine was used to cut a small hole in the patient's skull to treat seizures, headaches, or mental illness.

9th century

Medical literature from this period describes the use of an herb-soaked (soporific) sponge to anesthetize patients for surgery.

1842

Anesthesia use starts when Crawford W. Long performs the first surgery using ether, a flammable liquid.

1847

Ignaz Semmelweis discovers that contamination on surgeons' hands causes infections in postpartum women. He urges surgeons to wash hands between patients.

Don't worry. Surgical techniques have drastically improved over the years.

Surgery is the branch of medicine that treats disease, injury, and deformity using instruments or manual methods. Although it now involves sophisticated technology, the practice of surgery itself is nothing new. In fact, it dates back to ancient times.

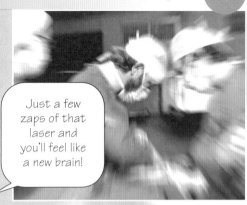

Just a few zaps of that laser and you'll feel like a new brain!

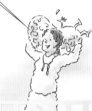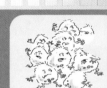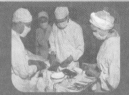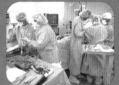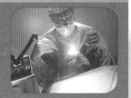

1863

The concept of nursing specialties arises when Florence Nightingale assigns separate areas for patients recovering from surgery.

1867

Modern surgical practices using aseptic technique begin when Joseph Lister pioneers the practice of hand and wound asepsis using carbolic acid.

1910

The American Nurses Association recommends that a registered nurse (RN) serve as circulating nurse and an RN or surgical technician serve as scrub nurse.

1940s

During World War II, the first recovery units are established to provide nursing care for patients after surgery.

1960s

Ambulatory surgery is performed for the first time, and ambulatory surgery programs are established.

1987

The use of laparoscopic surgery expands with introduction of laparoscopic cholecystectomy.

Early 1990s

Advances in endoscopy and video and laser technology lead to the development of minimally invasive surgery, which becomes the norm at the dawn of the 21st century.

See, didn't I tell you that would be a breeze?

Easy for you to say!

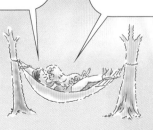

Surgical team

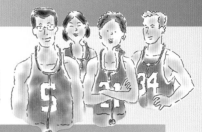

Preoperative team

Team member	Function
Preop nurse	▪ Performs the preoperative nursing assessment ▪ Prepares the patient for surgery
Physician, nurse practitioner, or physician's assistant	▪ Performs the preoperative history and physical examination
Clinical nurse specialist	▪ Collaborates with health care team members to deliver high-quality care to the surgical patient ▪ Participates in postoperative patient care

Operating room team

Sterile member	Function
Surgeon	▪ Performs the surgical procedure
Scrub nurse or technician	▪ Sets up special equipment, sterile table, and sutures ▪ Assists during the procedure and maintains the sterile surgical field
First assistant	▪ Assists the surgeon during the procedure
Nonsterile member	
Anesthesiologist	▪ Administers anesthesia and manages the patient's care during surgery and immediate postanesthesia phase
Nurse-anesthetist	▪ Administers anesthesia and monitors the patient during surgery
Circulating nurse	▪ Manages patient care and aseptic practices in the operating room (OR) ▪ Coordinates activities of OR personnel

Postoperative team

Team member	Function
Postanesthesia nurse	▪ Cares for the patient in the postanesthesia care unit (PACU) immediately after surgery
Medical-surgical or specialty unit nurse	▪ Provides postoperative care for the patient after discharge from the PACU

Informed consent

The surgical process typically starts in the surgeon's office, where the surgeon discusses the procedure with the patient and his family. Legally, the surgeon who will perform the procedure is responsible for explaining the procedure and its risks as well as for obtaining the patient's informed consent.

After the surgeon informs the patient about the procedure, he may ask you to obtain the patient's signature on the consent form. In this case, you would sign the form as a witness.

> By signing the consent form, the patient acknowledges that she understands the proposed procedure and its risks.

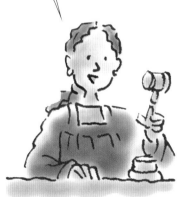

Sample consent form

Consent for operation and rendering of other medical services

1. I hereby authorize Dr. _Richards_ to perform upon _Ann Smith_ (Patient name) the following surgical and/or medical procedures: (State specific nature of the procedures to be performed) _Exploratory laparotomy_

2. I understand that the procedure(s) will be performed at Valley Medical Center by or under the supervision of D_. Richards_, who is authorized to utilize the services of other doctors members of the house staff as he or she de...

> The form should state the specific procedure under consideration.

3. It ha... ng the course of the operation, unforeseen c... ecessitate an extension of the original proced... an those set forth in Paragraph 1. I therefore authorize and request that the above named physician, and his or her associates or assistants, perform such medical or surgical procedures as are necessary and desirable in the exercise of professional judgment.

4. I understand the nature and purpose of the procedure(s), possible alternative methods of diagnosis or treatment, the risks involved, the possibility of complications, and the consequences of the procedure(s). I acknowledge that no guarantee or assurance has been made as to the results that may be obtained.

5. I authorize the above nam... regional anesthesia (for all other anes... nsent must be signed by the patient or pati...

> The patient acknowledges that she understands the procedure and its risks.

6. I understand that if it is nec... transfusion during this procedure or this hospitalization, the blood will be supplied by sources available to the hospital and tested in accordance with national and regional regulations. I understand that there are risks in transfusion, including but not limited to allergic, febrile, and hemolytic transfusion reactions and the transmission of infectious diseases, such as hepatitis and acquired immunodeficiency syndrome. I hereby consent to blood transfusion(s) and blood derivative(s).

7. I hereby authorize representatives from Valley Medical Center to photograph or videotape me for the purpose of research or medical education. It is understood and agreed that patient confi...

8. I authorize the physician named ab... and assistants and Valley Medical Center to ...s or to dispose of any tissue, organs, or othe... gery or other diagnostic procedures in accord... ractice.

> Signing means only that you've witnessed the patient's signature.

9. I certify that I have read and fully understand the above consent statement. In addition, I have been afforded an opportunity to ask whatever questions I might have regarding the procedure(s) to be performed and they have been answered to my satisfaction.

Ann Smith	_3/15/06_	_C. Gurney, RN_
Patient or Authorized Representative (State Relationship to Patient)	Date	Witness

If the patient is unable to consent on his or her own behalf, complete the following section:
Patient _____ is unable to consent because _____ .

_____
Legally Responsible Person

M. Richards, MD
Physician Obtaining Consent

Phases of surgery

Today, a patient can undergo a variety of procedures in an ambulatory surgery center and be discharged the same day.

More-complex surgical procedures still require post-operative hospitalization. Even if the patient will be hospitalized after the procedure, he's admitted to the hospital on the day of surgery, whereas in the past the patient was admitted to the hospital the evening before surgery.

Whether or not the patient is hospitalized, the surgical experience is divided into the preoperative, intraoperative, and postoperative phases.

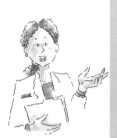

Preoperative phase

The preoperative phase starts with the patient's decision to have surgery and ends with her transfer to the OR. Care focuses on preparing and teaching the patient.

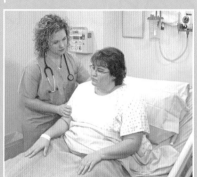

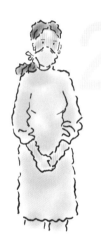

Intraoperative phase

The intraoperative phase starts when the patient is placed on the OR table and ends when she's transferred to the PACU. Care focuses on providing a safe environment during surgery.

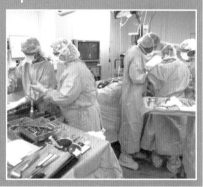

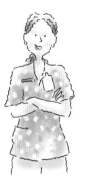

Postoperative phase

The postoperative phase starts when the patient is admitted to the PACU and ends when she no longer needs surgery-related nursing care. The focus is on preventing complications and relieving pain.

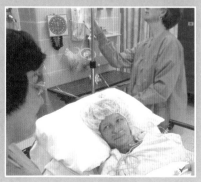

Diagnostic testing

Before surgery, the patient undergoes laboratory and diagnostic tests to provide baseline data and detect problems that could increase the risk of postoperative complications. For elective-surgery patients, tests are typically done in an outpatient setting during the week before surgery.

> The diagnostic tests performed depend on such factors as:
> ■ type of surgery scheduled
> ■ patient's age
> ■ preexisting medical conditions or risk factors.

Preoperative laboratory tests

- Blood typing and crossmatching
- Blood urea nitrogen and creatinine levels
- Coagulation studies
- Complete blood count (CBC)
- Electrolyte levels
- Human chorionic gonadotropin level
- Liver function studies
- Urinalysis

> Some patients may need to have preoperative laboratory tests, such as a CBC, or diagnostic studies, such as an ECG.

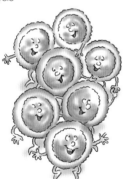
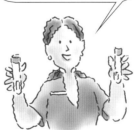

Diagnostic studies

- Chest X-ray
- Electrocardiogram (ECG)
- Pulmonary function tests

> Pseudocholinesterase deficiency places the patient at risk for prolonged respiratory paralysis when certain anesthetic agents are given.

Special tests

- ☑ Skeletal muscle biopsy (for patients at risk for malignant hyperthermia)
- ☑ Cholinesterase measurement (for patients at risk for pseudocholinesterase deficiency)

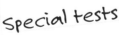
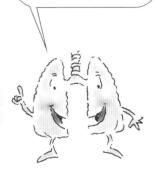

Preoperative assessment

A thorough preoperative nursing assessment helps to identify risk factors and establish a baseline for intraoperative and postoperative comparisons. During the assessment, focus on problem areas that the patient's history suggests and on body systems that surgery will directly affect.

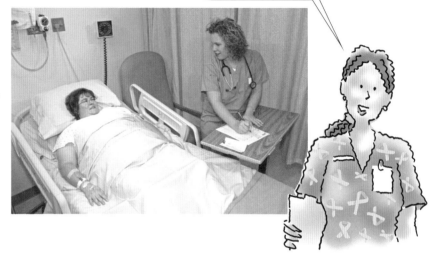

The health history is the main source of information about the patient's health and guides the physical examination.

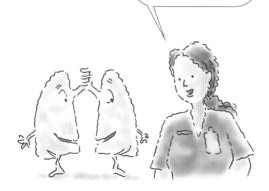

You're in good shape, but you're just one of many areas I'll need to check before the patient has surgery.

Surgical risk factors

- Pulmonary disorders, such as asthma or emphysema
- Cardiovascular disorders, such as hypertension, or a history of myocardial infarction
- Immobility
- Conditions that compromise health, such as malnutrition or immune deficiency
- Obesity
- Endocrine disorders, such as diabetes mellitus, hypothyroidism, or hyperthyroidism
- Fluid or electrolyte imbalances, such as hypovolemia, hypokalemia, or hyperkalemia
- Very young or very old age
- Coagulation disorders such as von Willebrand's disease

Health history

Biographical data

Name _____

Address _____

Date of birth (DOB) _____

Advance directive explained: ☐ Yes ☐ No

Living will on chart: ☐ Yes ☐ No

Name and phone numbers of two people to call, if necessary:

NAME   RELATIONSHIP   PHONE #

_____

_____

Chief complaint

History of present illness

_____

_____

Current medications

DRUG AND DOSE	FREQUENCY	LAST DOSE

Medical history

Allergies ☐ Tape ☐ Iodine ☐ Latex ☐ No known allergies

☐ Drug:_____

☐ Food: _____

☐ Environmental: _____

☐ Blood reaction: _____

☐ Other: _____

Be sure to include prescription drugs, over-the-counter drugs, herbal preparations, and vitamins and supplements.

Childhood illnesses

_____

_____

Previous hospitalizations

(illness, accident or injury, surgery, blood transfusion)

DATE

_____

_____

Health problems	Yes	No
Arthritis	☐	☐
Blood problem (anemia, sickle cell, clotting, bleeding)	☐	☐
Cancer	☐	☐
Diabetes mellitus	☐	☐
Eye problem (cataracts, glaucoma)	☐	☐
Heart disease (heart failure, MI, valve disease)	☐	☐
Hiatal hernia	☐	☐
HIV/AIDS	☐	☐
Hypertension	☐	☐
Kidney problem	☐	☐
Liver problem	☐	☐
Lung problem (asthma, bronchitis, emphysema, pneumonia, TB, shortness of breath)	☐	☐
Stroke	☐	☐
Thyroid problem	☐	☐
Ulcers (duodenal, peptic)	☐	☐
Psychological disorder	☐	☐

Obstetric history (females)

Last menstrual period (LMP) ____

Gravida _____ Para____

Menopause ☐ Yes ☐ No

Ask about the patient's feelings of safety to help identify physical, psychological, emotional, and sexual abuse issues.

Psychosocial history

Coping strategies

_____

Feelings of safety

_____

Smoker ☐ No ☐ Yes (# packs/day _____ # years _____)

Alcohol ☐ No ☐ Yes (type_____ amount/day_____)

Illicit drug use ☐ No ☐ Yes (type _____)

Religious and cultural observances

_____

Activities of daily living

Diet and exercise regimen_____

Elimination patterns _____

Sleep patterns _____

Work and leisure activities_____

Use of safety measures

(seat belt, bike helmet, sunscreen) _____

Ask about the patient's family medical history, including history of diabetes or heart disease.

Health maintenance history

Colonoscopy _____

Dental examination_____

Eye examination _____

Immunizations_____

Mammography _____

Family medical history

Health problem	Yes	No	Who (parent, grandparent, sibling)
Arthritis	☐	☐	_____
Cancer	☐	☐	_____
Diabetes mellitus	☐	☐	_____
Heart disease (heart failure, MI, valve disease)	☐	☐	_____
Hypertension	☐	☐	_____
Stroke	☐	☐	_____

Physical examination

The preoperative physical examination includes:

- general survey
- height and weight
- vital signs
- oxygen saturation
- head-to-toe assessment of major body systems.

Neurologic system

Assess the patient's level of consciousness, noting orientation to time, place, and person and ability to follow commands. Check pupillary reactions. Evaluate movement and sensation of the arms and legs.

Eyes, ears, nose, and throat

Assess the patient's vision, with and without corrective lenses. Evaluate his ability to hear spoken words clearly. Inspect the eyes and ears for discharge and nasal mucous membranes for dryness, irritation, and blood. Inspect the teeth, gums, and condition of the oral mucous membranes. Also palpate lymph nodes in the neck.

Respiratory system

Note respiratory rate and rhythm, and auscultate the patient's lung fields. Watch for flaring or retractions as the patient breathes. Inspect the lips, mucous membranes, and nail beds. Also inspect the sputum, noting its color, consistency, and other characteristics.

Cardiovascular system

Note the color and temperature of the patient's arms and legs, and assess the peripheral pulses. Check for edema and hair loss on the arms and legs. Also inspect the jugular veins and auscultate for heart sounds.

GI system

Auscultate for bowel sounds in all quadrants. Note abdominal distention or ascites. Gently palpate the abdomen for tenderness. Note whether the abdomen is soft, hard, or distended. Assess mucous membranes around the anus.

Musculoskeletal system

Assess the range of motion of major joints. Look for joint swelling, contractures, muscle atrophy, and obvious deformity. Evaluate muscle strength of the trunk, arms, and legs.

Genitourinary and reproductive systems

Note bladder distention or incontinence. If indicated, inspect the genitalia for rashes, edema, or deformity and, in a child, sexual maturity. (You may waive this inspection at the patient's request.) Also examine the breasts, noting abnormalities.

Integumentary system

Note sores, lesions, scars, pressure ulcers, rashes, bruises, discoloration, or petechiae. Also note skin turgor.

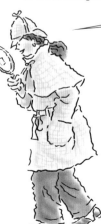

If you conduct a systematic body system review, you're much less likely to miss important clues.

Latex allergy screening

Latex is used in barrier protection products, surgical gloves, and medical equipment. Those at risk for latex allergy include people who have had multiple surgical procedures and people with a genetic predisposition to latex allergy. To find out if your patient is at risk for latex allergy, conduct a latex allergy screening.

Food allergy screening

Because certain foods may cause cross-sensitivity to latex, taking a food allergy history helps to screen for latex allergy. High-risk foods include avocados, bananas, and chestnuts. Moderate-risk foods include apples, carrots, celery, kiwi, melon, papaya, potatoes, and tomatoes.

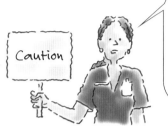

Caution

If your patient has a history of or is at high risk for latex allergy, follow your facility's policies and procedures to protect him. Be sure to alert the anesthesiologist and operating room staff.

Latex allergy screening questionnaire

Allergies

- Do you have a history of hay fever, asthma, eczema, allergies, or rashes? If so, what type of reaction have you experienced?
- Have you ever had an allergic reaction, local sensitivity, or itching after exposure to a latex product, such as a balloon or condom?
- Have you ever had shortness of breath or wheezing after blowing up a balloon or going to the dentist? Do you have itching in or around your mouth after eating a banana?
- If you've had shortness of breath or wheezing after blowing up a balloon, please describe your reaction.
- Are you allergic to any foods, especially avocados, bananas, chestnuts, or kiwi? If so, please describe your reaction.

Occupation

- What's your occupation?
- Are you exposed to latex at work?
- Have you had a reaction to latex products at work? If so, please describe your reaction.
- Have you ever noticed a rash on your hands after wearing latex gloves? If so, how soon after removing your gloves did the rash appear? What did it look like?

Personal history

- Do you have any congenital abnormalities? If so, please explain.
- Have you ever had itching, swelling, hives, cough, shortness of breath, or other allergy symptoms during or after using a condom or diaphragm or after a vaginal or rectal exam?

Surgical history

- Have you ever had surgery? If so, did you experience complications? Please describe them.
- Do you have spina bifida or a urinary tract problem that requires surgery or urinary catheterization?

Dental history

- Have you had dental procedures? If so, did complications result? Please describe them.

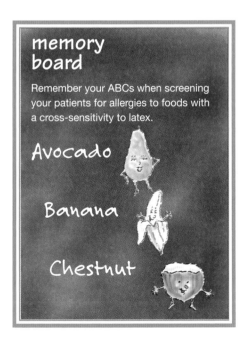

memory board

Remember your ABCs when screening your patients for allergies to foods with a cross-sensitivity to latex.

Avocado

Banana

Chestnut

Anesthesia evaluation

Preoperatively, a member of the anesthesia department sees every patient who's scheduled for anesthesia. The preanesthesia visit allows for assessment of the patient's physical status and emotional state.

The anesthesia evaluation includes a discussion of alternative anesthetic techniques and a review of the risks and benefits of these techniques, instruction on the importance of compliance with presurgery restrictions on food and fluids, and verification that the patient understands the anesthesia plans.

Make sure the evaluation has been completed before your patient goes into surgery.

Evaluating the airway

The anesthesiologist interviews the patient about past surgeries requiring endotracheal (ET) intubation and continues with an assessment of cervical spine mobility to determine any medical conditions or anatomic variations that may be associated with difficult ET intubation. Then he conducts a physical examination and evaluates the airway. One method used to classify the airway is the Mallampati airway classification system.

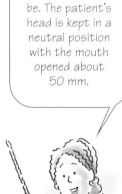

Classifying the airway predicts how difficult ET intubation will be. The patient's head is kept in a neutral position with the mouth opened about 50 mm.

Mallampati airway classification system

The Mallampati system has four classifications, based on the anatomic structures that can be visualized.

Class I	Class II	Class III	Class IV

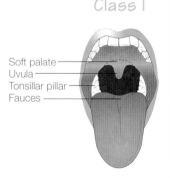
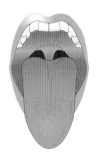
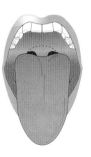
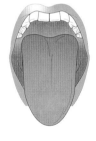

Soft palate
Uvula
Tonsillar pillar
Fauces

Soft palate, fauces, uvula, and both the anterior and posterior tonsillar pillars are visible.

Soft palate, fauces, and uvula are visible.

Only the soft palate and base of the uvula are visible.

Only the soft palate is visible.

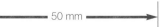

50 mm

Commonly used herbs that may interact with anesthetics

The anesthesiologist also reviews the patient's history of allergies and any currently used medications, herbal remedies, and supplements.

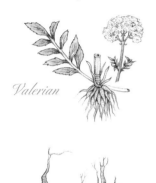

Valerian

Some herbs cause undesired effects when used with certain drugs. Usually, the patient should stop taking herbs at least 1 to 2 weeks before surgery.

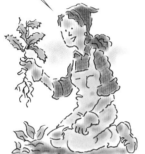

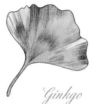

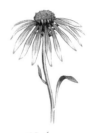

Ginkgo

Ginseng

Echinacea

Herbs that may interact with anesthetics include:
- chamomile
- echinacea
- feverfew
- flax
- garlic
- ginger
- ginkgo biloba
- ginseng
- goldenseal
- kava
- St. John's wort
- valerian.

ASA Physical Status Classification System

When the anesthesiologist has completed the anesthesia evaluation, he assigns the patient a numerical value according to the American Society of Anesthesiologists' (ASA) Physical Status Classification System. The higher the number assigned, the higher the patient's risk under anesthesia. An "E" beside the status designation denotes emergency surgery.

Knowledge of the ASA classification system helps the nurse anticipate and prepare for perioperative complications that may arise.

The higher the number, the greater the patient's risk under anesthesia.

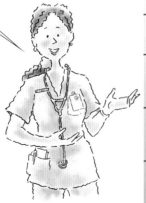

Classification	Description
P1	Normal, healthy patient
P2	Patient with mild systemic disease (such as controlled hypertension)
P3	Patient with severe systemic disease that limits activity (such as angina)
P4	Patient with severe systemic disease that poses a constant threat to life (such as heart failure or advanced pulmonary, renal, or hepatic dysfunction)
P5	Moribund patient not expected to survive without surgery (such as a patient with a ruptured abdominal aortic aneurysm)
P6	Patient declared brain-dead whose organs are being removed for donation

Patient teaching

Patient teaching at the preadmission and preoperative stages is crucial. Effective teaching helps the patient cope with the physical and psychological stress of surgery.

Adapt your teaching to the patient's age, understanding level, and cultural background. Also, clarify any misconceptions she has about surgery or hospitalization. Consider the needs of the family or caregiver, too.

Finally, be sure to evaluate the patient's understanding of your teaching.

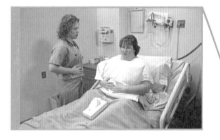

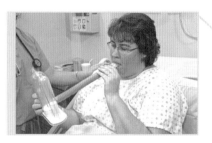

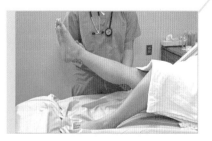

✔ Medications
✔ Diagnostic tests
✔ Dietary and fasting guidelines
✔ Surgical preparation
✔ Anesthesia concerns
✔ Surgical procedure
✔ PACU experience
✔ Pain control
✔ Coughing and deep-breathing exercises
✔ Spirometer use
✔ Postoperative exercises
✔ Use of assistive devices, such as crutches or a walker
✔ Postoperative tubes and drains

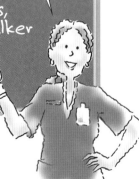

Be sure to cover these topics in your patient teaching.

Discharge planning

Start planning for discharge at your first contact with the patient. By recognizing potential problems early, you're more likely to have a successful discharge plan.

The initial nursing history and preoperative assessment, along with subsequent assessments, provide useful information for discharge planning. To ensure appropriate home care after discharge, include family members or other caregivers in the planning process.

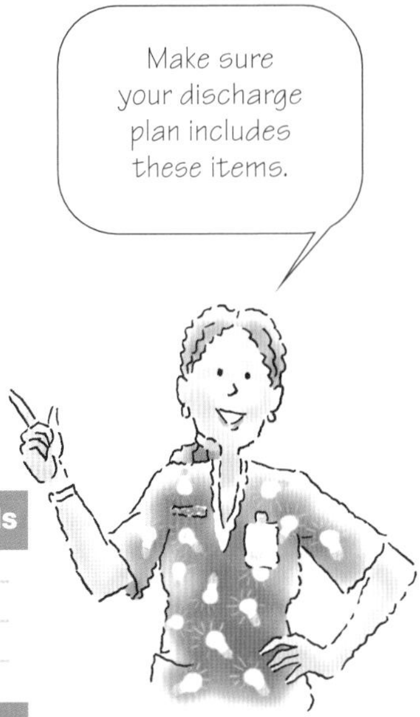

Make sure your discharge plan includes these items.

Discharge planning needs

Tailor the discharge plan to the patient's needs — including physiologic, psychological, and social factors and strengths as well as the patient's and his family's strengths and limitations.

Medications

Home care procedures and referrals

Recommended diet

Potential complications

Activity

Return appointments

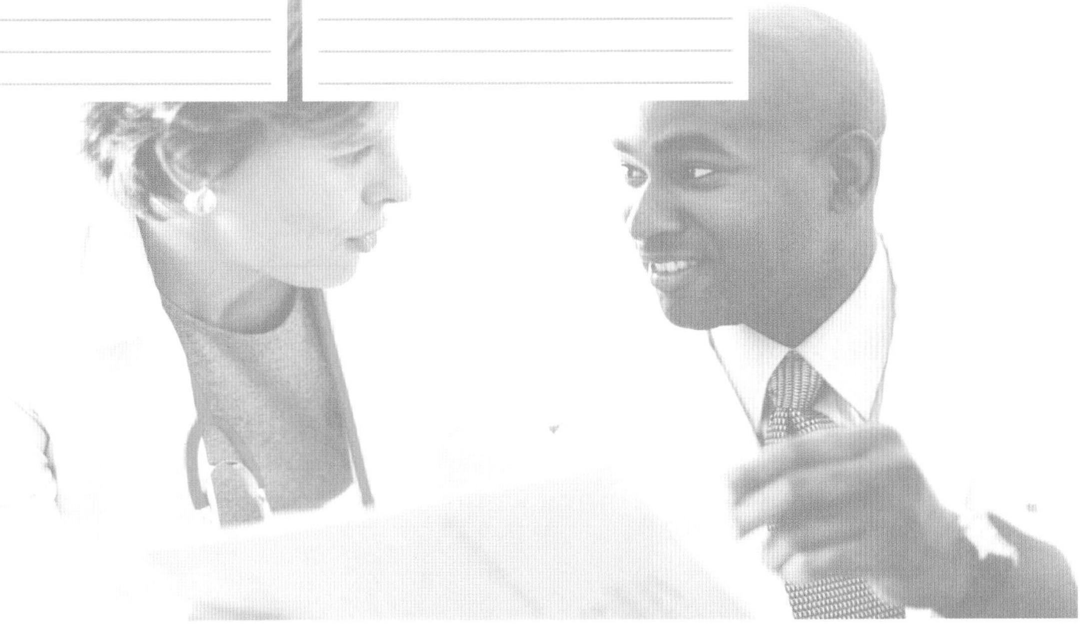

Preoperative verification

Preoperative verification ensures that all relevant patient documents and diagnostic test results are available and have been reviewed before surgery.

The Joint Commission on Accreditation of Healthcare Organizations (JCAHO) has established a universal protocol to prevent wrong-person, wrong-site, and wrong-procedure surgery. Confirming the patient's identity prevents wrong-person surgery. Marking the surgical site prevents wrong-site surgery. Using a preoperative checklist prevents wrong-procedure surgery.

According to JCAHO, acceptable patient identifiers include:
- patient's name
- assigned identification number
- date of birth
- Social Security number
- address
- photograph
- other person-specific identifiers.

Each facility chooses two patient identifiers. Make sure you know which two your facility uses.

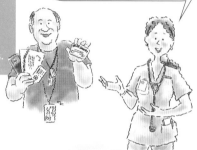

Op sight

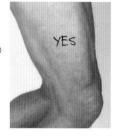

Marking the surgical site

Marking the surgical site ensures that the procedure is being carried out on the correct anatomic site. JCAHO requires each facility to implement a protocol for marking the exact site of any operative or invasive procedure involving:
- right or left distinction
- multiple structures, such as fingers and toes
- multiple levels, such as procedures involving the spine.

The site should be marked before the patient is taken to the area where the procedure will be performed. It should be marked with a marker that doesn't wash off when the site is prepared.

JCAHO recommends that the person who performs the procedure mark the site. The patient or whoever has authority to provide informed consent should be involved in the marking process.

The marking must be visible after the patient has been prepared and draped for the procedure.

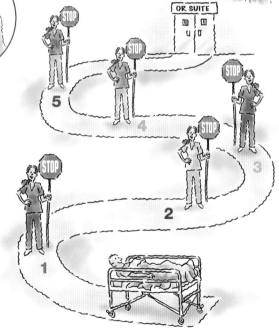

Checkpoint key

1 Correct patient identification?
2 Correct procedure side or site?
3 Team agreement on procedure?
4 Implants available (if needed)?
5 Special equipment or requirements available (if needed)?

Preoperative checklist and surgical identification form

Instructions: All items checked "No" require follow-up. Follow-up is to be documented in the "Additional information/Comments" section until resolved.

Patient name: Zacher, Timothy   Medical record number: 987654

Preop checklist	Yes	No	Resolved	Initials
ID band on	✓			NRC
Allergies noted/Bracelet	✓			NRC
History and Physical (present and reviewed)	✓			NRC
"Surgical Informed Consent" signed	✓			NRC
"Anesthesia Informed Consent" signed	✓			NRC
Preop teaching	✓			NRC
Prep, as ordered	✓			NRC
NPO after midnight	✓			NRC
Dentures, capped teeth, cosmetics, glasses, contact lenses, wig removed	N/A			
Voided/Catheter inserted	✓			NRC
Medical clearance/Physician's name	✓			NRC
TEDS, as ordered	N/A			
SCD, as ordered	N/A			
PCA teaching, as ordered	✓			NRC
Type and Cross/Screen drawn (if ordered must have "Blood Informed Consent" signed)	N/A			
"Blood Informed Consent" signed	N/A			
Lab results on chart	✓			NRC
ECG on chart	✓			NRC
Chest X-ray on chart	✓			NRC

Abnormal results reported to H&H   Dr. Schoblitz
Date and time 4/28/06 0800   Reported by NRC
Temp. 98.6   Pulse 84   Resp. 18   B/P 132/82
Valuables destination: ☑ To safe ☐ To family (name) _____
X Norma R. Clay, RN   NRC
RN's signature   Initials
X _____
Transferring RN's signature   Date   Time
Additional information/Comments:

Surgical patient identification form

Nursing Floor RN Patient Identification
☑ Patient ID bracelet personally observed
☑ Patient questioned verbally regarding ID, Procedure, and Site
☑ Patient's chart reviewed to verify ID, Procedure, and Site
X Norma R. Clay, RN   4/28/06   0800
RN's signature   Date   Time

Preop Anesthesia Patient Identification
☐ Patient ID bracelet personally observed
☐ Patient questioned verbally regarding ID, Procedure, and Site
☐ Patient's chart reviewed to verify ID, Proc
X _____
Anesthesiologist/Anesthetist's signature   Date

Operating Room and Anesthesia Personnel Patient Identification
Operative Procedure and Site
ANES CIRC Nurse
☐ ☐ Patient ID bracelet person
☐ ☐ Patient questioned verbally Procedure, and Site
☐ ☐ Patient's chart reviewed to Procedure, and Site
☐ ☐ Surgical site confirmed
☐ ☐ Time-out performed
X _____
Anesthesiologist/Anesthetist's signature   Time
X _____
CIRC Nurse's signature

Surgeon's Patient Identification Statement
☐ Patient ID bracelet personally observed
☐ Patient questioned verbally regarding ID, Procedure, and Site
☐ Surgical site marked
X _____
Surgeon's signature

> Before the patient leaves your unit for the OR, check to make sure that all of these important steps have been done.

Taking a "time-out"

The health care team should take a "time-out" in the location where the procedure will be done—just before the procedure starts—for final verification of the right patient, right site, and right procedure. The "time-out" should include verifying correct patient positioning and availability of implants or special equipment needed for the procedure.

If only one person is involved in the procedure (as in some bedside procedures), that person must take a brief "time-out" to confirm the correct patient, site, and procedure. Always document that a "time-out" was taken.

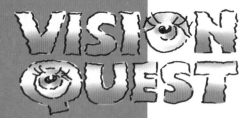

Picture imperfect

Identify this patient's six surgical risk factors.

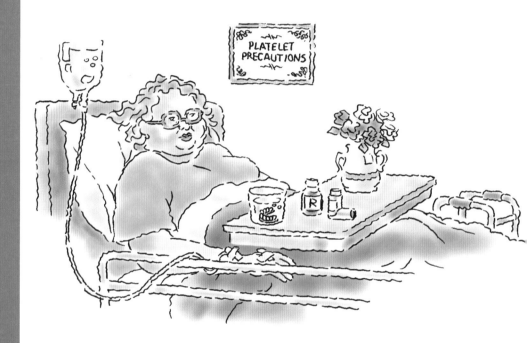

1. _____

2. _____

3. _____

4. _____

5. _____

6. _____

Answers: Picture imperfect 1. Advanced age, 2. Obesity, 3. Immobility (represented by the walker), 4. Endocrine problem (diabetes, represented by the insulin vial on the overbed table), 5. Coagulation disorder (represented by the "Platelet precautions" sign above the bed), 6. Pulmonary disorder (asthma, represented by the inhaler on the overbed table).

2
Fundamentals of anesthesia

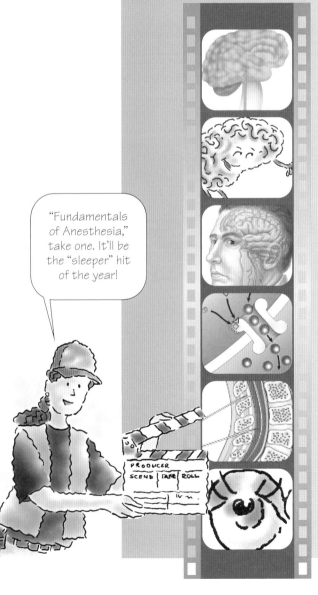

"Fundamentals of Anesthesia," take one. It'll be the "sleeper" hit of the year!

- Anesthesia basics 20
- General anesthesia stages 21
- Balanced anesthesia 23
- Four levels of sedation and anesthesia 24
- General anesthetics 25
- Regional anesthetics 36
- Local anesthetics 37
- Vision quest 38

Anesthesia basics

Anesthesia is an artificially induced state of partial or total sensation loss in which the patient doesn't feel pain. Without it, surgeons wouldn't be able to perform most types of surgery because patients couldn't tolerate the pain and the body's physiologic response to pain would cause hemodynamic instability.

Understanding pain transmission

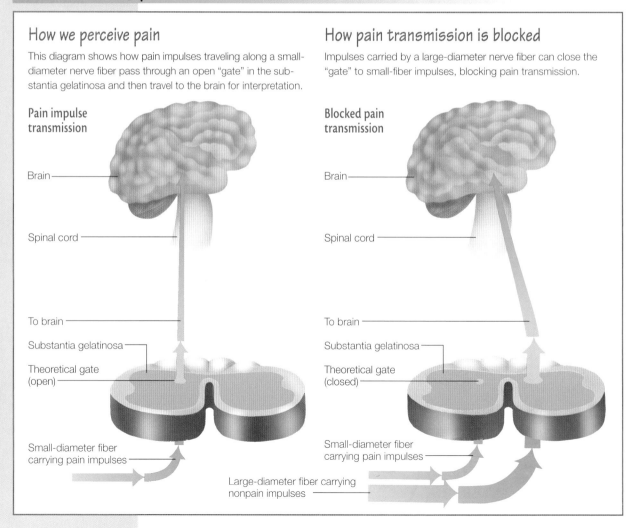

How we perceive pain

This diagram shows how pain impulses traveling along a small-diameter nerve fiber pass through an open "gate" in the substantia gelatinosa and then travel to the brain for interpretation.

Pain impulse transmission

Brain

Spinal cord

To brain

Substantia gelatinosa

Theoretical gate (open)

Small-diameter fiber carrying pain impulses

How pain transmission is blocked

Impulses carried by a large-diameter nerve fiber can close the "gate" to small-fiber impulses, blocking pain transmission.

Blocked pain transmission

Brain

Spinal cord

To brain

Substantia gelatinosa

Theoretical gate (closed)

Small-diameter fiber carrying pain impulses

Large-diameter fiber carrying nonpain impulses

Goals of general anesthesia

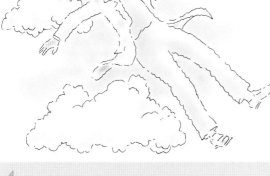

The goals of general anesthesia include...causing unconsciousness and...providing... Ohhh...I'm getting so sleepy...

Types of anesthesia

- General
- Regional (spinal and epidural)
- Local

The anesthesiologist consults with the surgeon and patient to decide which type of anesthesia or sedation to use. The choice depends on:

- type, location, and duration of surgery
- technical intricacy of the procedure
- patient's age and physical condition
- patient's previous anesthetic history
- anesthesiologist's personal preference, expertise, and clinical judgment.

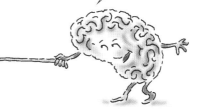

She's completely under now. Here are the goals she was starting to tell you about.

1 To cause loss of consciousness

2 To prevent or reduce pain (providing analgesia)

3 To eliminate normal reflexes

4 To relax skeletal muscles

5 To cause amnesia (blocking memory of the procedure)

6 To maintain physiologic stability

General anesthesia stages

General anesthesia consists of four stages; however, the patient normally proceeds through three stages—analgesia, excitement, and surgical anesthesia—marked by defined physiologic changes in his respiration, oculomotor reflexes, pharyngeal and laryngeal reflexes, and muscle tone. Stage four, medullary depression, indicates overdose and ends in circulatory collapse.

In addition, stage III—the surgical anesthesia stage—has four separate planes:

- Plane 1—regular respirations, rapid side-to-side eye movement, and abolished lid reflex
- Plane 2—fixation of eyes and decreased intercostal muscle activity
- Plane 3—complete intercostal muscle paralysis
- Plane 4—complete cessation of spontaneous respiration.

Stages of anesthesia

The original stages of anesthesia were based on the use of ether and chloroform, neither of which is used today. Modern anesthetic agents have different properties but are still compared to the classic anesthesia stages.

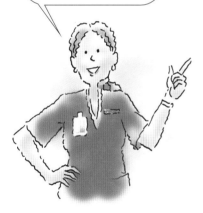

With anesthetic agents used today, the patient passes rapidly through stage II — the excitement stage — with less-frequent involuntary activity.

Anesthesia stage	Respiration		Ocular movements
	INTERCOSTAL	DIAPHRAGM	
Stage I (analgesia)			Voluntary control
Stage II (excitement)			
Stage III (surgical anesthesia) Plane 1			
Plane 2			
Plane 3			
Plane 4			
Stage IV (medullary depression)			

Note: Wedge points indicate when the signs and reflexes disappear.

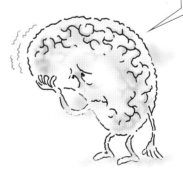

Stage IV — the medullary depression stage — should never be reached! Apnea occurs, followed by circulatory and respiratory collapse and even death.

Pupil size (NO PREMEDICATION)	Eye reflexes	Pharynx/larynx reflexes	Lacrimation	Muscle tone
			Normal	Normal
				Tense struggle
	Lid tone	Swallow / Retch / Vomit		
	Corneal	Glottis		
	Pupillary light reflex			
		Carinal		

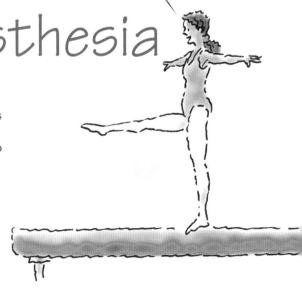

For balanced anesthesia, the patient receives a combination of agents. This rapidly induces anesthesia and causes sleep, analgesia, muscle relaxation, and reflex elimination with minimal undesired effects.

Balanced anesthesia

In balanced anesthesia, a combination of anesthetic agents is given in doses sufficient to cause optimal desired effects but with minimal undesired effects. Typically, the patient receives an I.V. agent (barbiturate, nonbarbiturate, benzodiazepine, opioid, or muscle relaxant) followed by an inhalation agent to rapidly induce anesthesia.

To maintain anesthesia, the patient may receive a mixture of a volatile anesthetic (delivered through an endotracheal [ET] tube by an anesthesia machine), nitrous oxide, oxygen, and titrated doses of one or more I.V. agents.

Four levels of sedation and anesthesia

The Joint Commission on Accreditation of Healthcare Organizations defines four levels of sedation and anesthesia, which apply when the patient receives general or regional anesthesia or moderate or deep sedation. Keep in mind that some drugs used to induce general anesthesia can be given in lower doses to produce sedation.

With minimal sedation (anxiolysis), the patient responds normally to verbal commands. Cognitive function and coordination may be impaired, but ventilatory and cardiovascular functions are intact.

With moderate sedation or moderate analgesia, consciousness is decreased but the patient responds purposefully to verbal commands (or to verbal commands with light tactile stimulation). He has adequate spontaneous ventilation, can maintain a patent airway on his own, and maintains cardiovascular function.

With deep sedation or deep analgesia, the level of consciousness decreases. Although the patient responds purposefully to repeated tactile or painful stimuli, he can't be aroused easily. His ventilatory function may be impaired, and he may need assistance to maintain a patent airway. Usually, cardiovascular function remains normal.

In general anesthesia, the patient loses consciousness and can't be aroused even with painful stimuli. He usually needs assistance to maintain a patent airway and may need positive-pressure ventilation because his spontaneous ventilation or neuromuscular function is depressed. Cardiovascular function may be impaired.

Orca

1 The first stop on my dive is the minimal sedation level, where the patient maintains normal breathing and cardiovascular function.

2 According to my depth gauge, I'm now at the moderate sedation level.

3 This is called the deep sedation or deep analgesia state.

4 Now I'm at the deepest level — general anesthesia. Better check my dive table to see how long I can stay down here!

General anesthetics

Drugs used for general anesthesia include inhalation agents and a wide range of I.V. drugs.

Inhalation agents

Inhalation anesthetics are gases or vapors delivered through the respiratory tract (typically through an ET tube or mask). They're used to induce or maintain anesthesia.

Inhalation agents work mainly by depressing the central nervous system (CNS). This causes unconsciousness, relaxes muscles, and makes the patient unresponsive to pain and other sensory stimulation. These agents also impair respiratory and circulatory function, depress the myocardium, and may impair renal or hepatic function.

Rarely, hepatotoxicity develops a few days after halothane use in adults — most commonly after multiple drug exposures. Symptoms include rash, fever, jaundice, nausea, vomiting, eosinophilia, and liver function changes.

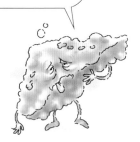

Depressant effects of inhalation agents

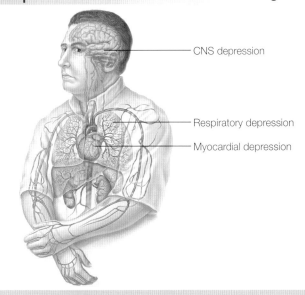

- CNS depression
- Respiratory depression
- Myocardial depression

Inhalation agents	Indications	Adverse reactions	Nursing considerations
Inorganic gas ■ nitrous oxide **Volatile agents** ■ desflurane (Suprane) ■ enflurane (Ethrane) ■ halothane (Fluothane) ■ isoflurane (Forane) ■ sevoflurane (Ultane)	Inhalation agents are used to induce and maintain general anesthesia.	■ Exaggerated response to normal dose ■ Respiratory and myocardial depression ■ Confusion ■ Sedation ■ Nausea ■ Vomiting ■ Arrhythmias ■ Hypothermia	■ Provide humidified supplemental oxygen during the recovery phase, as ordered. ■ Postoperatively, monitor the patient for respiratory depression, CNS depression, and arrhythmias.

I.V. agents

I.V. drugs are commonly combined with inhalants to cause unconsciousness, analgesia, and muscle relaxation. They promote rapid anesthesia induction and are used in balanced anesthesia. For surgery requiring only brief anesthesia, such as outpatient surgery, I.V. drugs may be used alone.

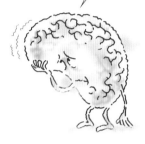

I feel so groggy. I think my reticular activating system needs a jump start.

Barbiturates

Barbiturates make CNS neurons less excitable and enhance response to the neurotransmitter gamma-aminobutyric acid, or GABA for short. This effect inhibits the stimulation response of the reticular activating system (RAS) — the area of the brain that controls alertness.

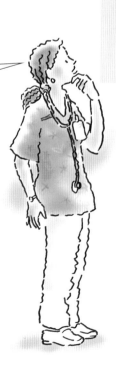

Even though barbiturates are short acting, it's important to monitor your patient postoperatively to avoid complications.

Barbiturates	Indications	Adverse reactions	Nursing considerations
▪ methohexital (Brevital) ▪ thiopental sodium (Pentothal)	Barbiturates are used to induce general anesthesia.	▪ Respiratory depression ▪ Cough ▪ Hiccups ▪ Muscle twitching ▪ Laryngo-spasm	▪ Postoperatively, monitor the patient for respiratory depression, CNS depression, and arrhythmias. ▪ Stay alert for laryngo-spasm, airway obstruction, hypoxemia, and respiratory depression. ▪ Barbiturates have no analgesic properties.

Nonbarbiturates

Like barbiturates, nonbarbiturates enhance the brain's response to GABA and reduce its response to RAS stimulation.

Nonbarbiturates	Indications	Adverse reactions	Nursing considerations
▪ etomidate (Amidate) ▪ propofol (Diprivan)	▪ Etomidate and propofol are used to induce general anesthesia. ▪ Propofol is also used to maintain general anesthesia.	▪ Profound respiratory depression (with propofol) ▪ Cough ▪ Hiccups ▪ Muscle twitching	▪ Be prepared to provide airway support. ▪ Propofol has no analgesic properties but may have some antiemetic properties. ▪ Stay alert for complaints of pain at the injection site.

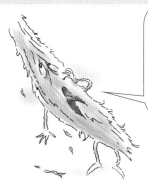

I keep twitching! They tell me it's an adverse effect of nonbarbiturates. But it could just be all that coffee I drank this morning...

Dissociative agents

The dissociative agent ketamine (Ketalar) acts directly on the cortex and limbic system of the brain, producing a profound sense of dissociation from the environment. Ketamine produces hallucinogenic effects and, for this reason, is rarely given to adults or adolescents.

Dissociative agent	Indications	Adverse reactions	Nursing considerations
ketamine (Ketalar)	Ketamine is used for short diagnostic and surgical procedures that don't require muscle relaxants.	▪ Increased salivation ▪ Delirium ▪ Hallucinations ▪ Disorientation ▪ Excitement ▪ Hypertension ▪ Tachycardia ▪ Increased intracranial pressure	▪ Monitor for increased oral secretions and be prepared to provide airway support. ▪ Ketamine causes hallucinations, unpleasant dreams, and delirium during recovery, especially in patients between puberty and age 65. ▪ Ketamine also reduces tactile and auditory stimulation during the recovery phase.

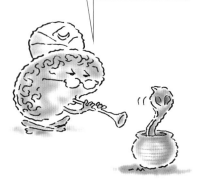

Either I'm delirious from the ketamine, or I'm a snake charmer in full swami regalia.

Benzodiazepines

Like barbiturates and nonbarbiturates, benzodiazepines enhance the brain's response to GABA and reduce its response to RAS stimulation.

Benzodiazepines	Indications	Adverse reactions	Nursing considerations
▪ diazepam (Valium) ▪ midazolam (Versed)	▪ Benzodiazepines are used to induce general anesthesia. ▪ Midazolam is also used to maintain general anesthesia and for moderate sedation.	▪ CNS and respiratory depression (especially when given with opioids) ▪ Drowsiness ▪ Confusion ▪ Ataxia ▪ Weakness ▪ Dizziness ▪ Nystagmus ▪ Vertigo ▪ Fainting ▪ Dysarthria ▪ Headache ▪ Tremor ▪ Glassy-eyed appearance	▪ Be prepared to provide airway support. ▪ An older adult may experience increased sedation, dizziness, and confusion (especially with diazepam). Take steps to ensure patient safety. ▪ Midazolam is the preferred drug because its half-life is much shorter than that of diazepam.

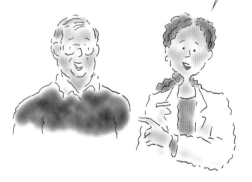

When given diazepam, older patients are at risk for increased sedation, dizziness, and confusion.

How benzodiazepines work

These illustrations show how benzodiazepines work at the cellular level.

Speed and passage

The number of chloride ions in the postsynaptic neuron affects the speed of impulses from a presynaptic neuron across the synapse. Passage of chloride ions into the postsynaptic neuron depends on gamma-aminobutyric acid (GABA), an inhibitory neurotransmitter.

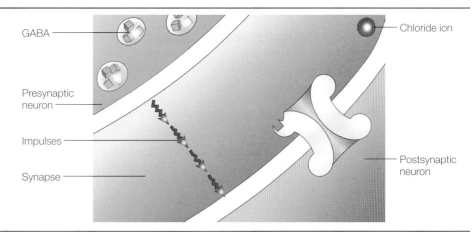

GABA

Presynaptic neuron

Impulses

Synapse

Chloride ion

Postsynaptic neuron

A binding proposition

When released from the presynaptic neuron, GABA travels across the synapse and binds to GABA receptors on the postsynaptic neuron. This binding opens chloride channels, in turn allowing chloride ions to flow into the postsynaptic neuron and slowing nerve impulses.

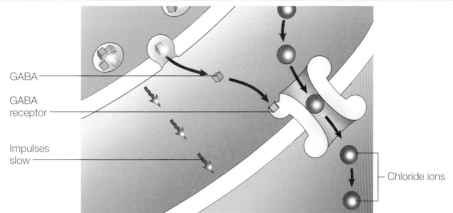

GABA

GABA receptor

Impulses slow

Chloride ions

Impulses at an impasse

Benzodiazepines bind to receptors on or near the GABA receptor, enhancing GABA effects and letting more chloride ions flow into the postsynaptic neuron. This depresses nerve impulses, causing them to slow or even stop.

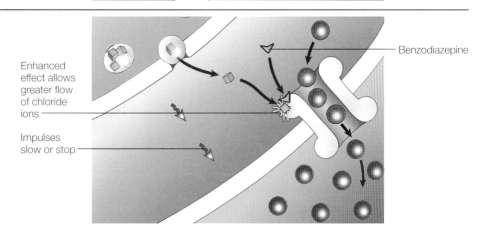

Enhanced effect allows greater flow of chloride ions

Impulses slow or stop

Benzodiazepine

Opioids

Opioids work by occupying sites on specialized receptors throughout the CNS and by modifying neurotransmitter release from sensory nerves entering the CNS. Opioids have analgesic properties and are used to manage surgical pain.

> Be on the lookout for respiratory depression after administering an opioid.

Opioids	Indications	Adverse reactions	Nursing considerations
▪ alfentanil (Alfenta) ▪ fentanyl (Sublimaze) ▪ morphine ▪ sufentanil (Sufenta)	▪ Opioids are used to induce and maintain general anesthesia. ▪ They're also used for moderate sedation and to manage pain.	▪ CNS depression ▪ Respiratory depression and hypoventilation ▪ Bronchoconstriction ▪ Arrhythmias ▪ Skeletal muscle and chest wall rigidity (with fentanyl)	▪ Postoperatively, monitor the patient for CNS depression, respiratory depression, and arrhythmias. ▪ Be sure to keep emergency equipment at hand.

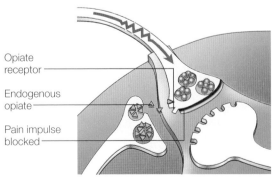

How opioids control pain

Morphine and other opioid agonists control pain by mimicking the body's natural pain control mechanisms.

Where neurons meet

In the spinal cord's dorsal horn, peripheral pain neurons meet central nervous system (CNS) neurons. At the synapse, the pain neuron releases substance P, a pain neurotransmitter. This substance helps transfer pain impulses to the CNS neurons that carry those impulses to the brain.

Taking up space

In theory, spinal interneurons respond to stimulation from descending neurons by releasing endogenous opiates. These opiates bind to peripheral pain neurons to inhibit substance P release and slow pain impulse transmission.

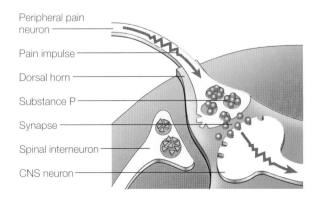

Peripheral pain neuron
Pain impulse
Dorsal horn
Substance P
Synapse
Spinal interneuron
CNS neuron

Opiate receptor
Endogenous opiate
Pain impulse blocked

Opioid and benzodiazepine reversal agents

Reversal agents are used during surgery or postoperatively in case the unwanted effects of benzodiazepines or opioids need to be reversed. Naloxone (Narcan) reverses the CNS and respiratory depressant effects of opioids by occupying opiate receptor sites, displacing opioids attached to these receptors and preventing opioids from binding at these sites.

Flumazenil (Romazicon) reverses the CNS effects of benzodiazepines by binding at benzodiazepine receptor sites.

Reversal agents	Indications	Adverse reactions	Nursing considerations
naloxone (Narcan)	Naloxone is used to reverse the effects of opioids.	▪ Arrhythmias ▪ Hypertension ▪ Noncardiogenic pulmonary edema ▪ Seizures ▪ Tachycardia ▪ Tremors	▪ Reversal agents have a shorter duration than opioids and benzodiazepines, so stay alert for recurrent respiratory and CNS depression. ▪ Repeated doses of the reversal agent may be needed. ▪ Keep emergency equipment at hand. ▪ Be aware that abrupt opioid or benzodiazepine reversal in chronic users of these drugs may cause withdrawal symptoms, such as CNS excitement, agitation, arrhythmias, diaphoresis, nausea, vomiting, hypertension, and tachycardia.
flumazenil (Romazicon)	Flumazenil is used to reverse the effects of benzodiazepines.	▪ Arrhythmias ▪ Agitation ▪ Blurred vision ▪ Seizures	

> Someone throw me a life preserver! Naloxone can cause pulmonary edema — not to mention some other scary adverse reactions.

Stopping substance P

Opioids supplement this pain-blocking effect by binding with free opiate receptors to inhibit substance P release. They also alter consciousness of pain, although how this mechanism works remains unknown.

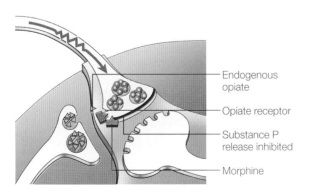

Endogenous opiate

Opiate receptor

Substance P release inhibited

Morphine

Neuromuscular blocking agents

During some surgical procedures, muscle tone must be controlled. To achieve this effect, neuromuscular blocking agents (muscle relaxants) may be given. These drugs relax skeletal muscles by disrupting nerve impulse transmission at the motor endplate. They also promote smooth-muscle relaxation.

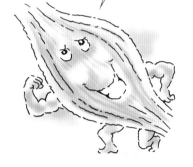

Neuromuscular blocking agents can be either depolarizing or nondepolarizing.

How the depolarizing neuromuscular blocker works

The only therapeutic depolarizing neuromuscular blocker, succinylcholine mimics the action of acetylcholine and binds to cholinergic receptor sites on skeletal muscle cells. This causes the cells to depolarize, leading to muscle relaxation.

Succinylcholine metabolizes rapidly, but at a slower rate than acetylcholine. Thus, the drug stays attached to receptor sites on skeletal muscle membranes for a long time, preventing motor endplate repolarization. As long as the cells stay depolarized, they can't respond to further acetylcholine stimulation. As a result, nerve impulse transmission at the motor endplates is disrupted, causing neuromuscular blockade.

How nondepolarizing neuromuscular blockers work

Nondepolarizing neuromuscular blockers compete with acetylcholine at cholinergic receptor sites on skeletal muscle cell membranes. This competition prevents acetylcholine from reaching the motor endplate, thus disrupting nerve impulse transmission at the endplate, resulting in neuromuscular blockade.

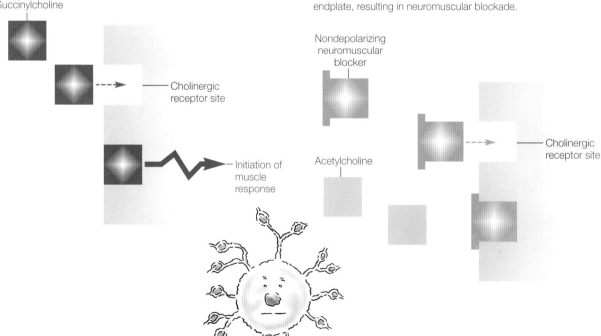

Succinylcholine

Cholinergic receptor site

Initiation of muscle response

Nondepolarizing neuromuscular blocker

Acetylcholine

Cholinergic receptor site

Neuromuscular blocking agents	Indications	Adverse reactions	Nursing considerations
Depolarizing • succinylcholine (Anectine)	• Succinylcholine is used to provide skeletal muscle relaxation as a component of general anesthesia. • It's also the drug of choice for short-term skeletal muscle relaxation for ET intubation.	• Prolonged apnea • Respiratory depression • Hypotension • Arrhythmias • Fasciculations	• Prior to postoperative extubation, be sure to assess respiratory function and muscle strength. • Some antibiotics (including aminoglycosides, vancomycin, tetracycline, and bacitracin) may prolong the neuromuscular blockade. • Succinylcholine is contraindicated in patients with a personal or family history of malignant hyperthermia or pseudocholinesterase deficiency as well as in patients with acute angle-closure glaucoma. • Be aware that succinylcholine shouldn't be used in patients with severe trauma, burns, or hyperkalemia.
Nondepolarizing • atracurium (Tracrium) • cisatracurium (Nimbex) • doxacurium (Nuromax) • mivacurium (Mivacron) • pancuronium • rocuronium (Zemuron) • tubocurarine (D-tubocurarine, Curare) • vecuronium (Norcuron)	• Nondepolarizing neuromuscular blockers are used to provide skeletal muscle relaxation as a component of general anesthesia. • They're also used to provide short-term skeletal muscle relaxation during ET intubation.	• Apnea • Respiratory depression • Hypotension • Bronchospasm • Excessive bronchial and salivary secretions • Skin reactions • Tachycardia, arrhythmias, and hypertension (with pancuronium)	• Prior to postoperative extubation, be sure to assess respiratory function and muscle strength. • Some antibiotics (including aminoglycosides, vancomycin, tetracycline, and bacitracin) may prolong neuromuscular blockade. • Nondepolarizing neuromuscular blocking agents may be reversed with anticholinesterase drugs. • Prior to reversal, you must assess the adequacy of recovery from the nondepolarizing blocking agent.

Respirations must be supported after administration of neuromuscular blocking agents.

Nondepolarizing neuromuscular blocker reversal agents

Anticholinesterase drugs block the action of acetylcholinesterase at cholinergic receptor sites. This effect prevents acetylcholine from breaking down and allows it to build up at the motor endplate. Acetylcholine then displaces the nondepolarizing neuromuscular blocker and restores normal neuromuscular transmission.

An anticholinergic drug (such as atropine or glycopyrrolate) is given with anticholinesterases to prevent certain adverse effects. Anticholinergics interrupt parasympathetic nerve impulses in the CNS and autonomic nervous system and prevent acetylcholine from stimulating muscarine receptors (a type of cholinergic receptor).

Reversal agents	Indications	Adverse reactions	Nursing considerations
Anticholinesterase drugs • edrophonium (Tensilon, Enlon) • neostigmine (Prostigmin) • pyridostigmine (Regonol)	• Anticholinesterase drugs are used to reverse the effects of nondepolarizing neuromuscular blocking agents.	• Bradycardia • Bronchoconstriction • Excessive salivation • Hypotension	• Before anticholinesterase administration, evaluate the patient's respiratory function and muscle strength in order to assess adequacy of recovery from the neuromuscular blockade. • To determine if the patient is ready for anticholinesterase administration, use peripheral nerve stimulation to assess the degree of blockade. • Be aware that anticholinesterase drugs are given with an anticholinergic. Short-acting edrophonium is always given with atropine (not with the slower-acting glycopyrrolate).
Anticholinergic drugs • atropine • glycopyrrolate (Robinul)	• Anticholinergic drugs are given with anticholinesterase drugs to prevent the muscarinic effects of the reversal. • They may be given preoperatively to decrease secretions. • Atropine is used to treat symptomatic bradycardia during surgery or postoperatively.	• Ataxia • Blurred vision • Bradycardia (paradoxical slowing of the heart rate with adult dose of atropine less than 0.5 mg) • Delirium • Dry mouth • Tachycardia • Urine retention	• Monitor the patient for arrhythmias. • Use atropine cautiously in patients with myocardial ischemia. • Atropine isn't recommended for patients with type 2 second-degree atrioventricular (AV) block or third-degree AV block. Also, it's contraindicated in patients with acute angle-closure glaucoma or obstructive uropathy.

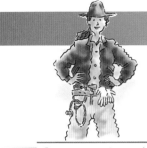

Train-of-four stimulation

Train-of-four is the most common peripheral nerve stimulation test used to monitor neuromuscular blockade in a patient receiving a neuromuscular blocker.

The peripheral nerve stimulator (shown below) delivers a small electric stimulus. The level of neuromuscular blockade is determined by observing the number of muscle twitches after stimulation. No twitch indicates that 100% of the nerve receptors are blocked, which exceeds the desired level of neuromuscular blockade. Two twitches out of four indicates neuromuscular blockade of roughly 85%.

The chart below shows the neuromuscular blockade level as indicated by the number of twitches.

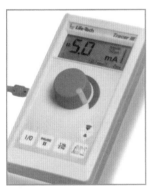

Number of twitches	Nerve receptors blocked
0 of 4	100%
1 of 4	90%
2 of 4	85%
3 of 4	80%
4 of 4	75% or less

How atropine speeds the heart rate

To understand how atropine affects the heart, first consider how the heart's electrical conduction system works.

Without the drug

When the neurotransmitter acetylcholine is released, the vagus nerve stimulates both the sinoatrial (SA) node (the heart's pacemaker) and the atrioventricular (AV) node, which controls conduction between the heart's atria and ventricles. This stimulation inhibits electrical conduction and slows the heart rate.

With the drug

Atropine competes with acetylcholine for cholinergic receptor sites on the SA and AV nodes. By blocking acetylcholine, atropine makes the heart beat faster.

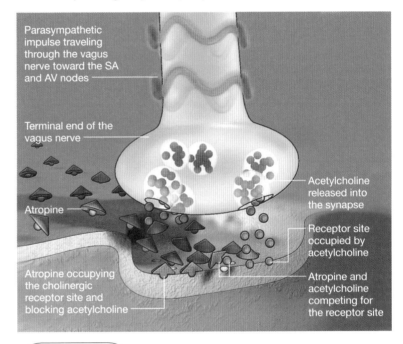

Parasympathetic impulse traveling through the vagus nerve toward the SA and AV nodes

Terminal end of the vagus nerve

Atropine

Atropine occupying the cholinergic receptor site and blocking acetylcholine

Acetylcholine released into the synapse

Receptor site occupied by acetylcholine

Atropine and acetylcholine competing for the receptor site

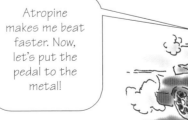

Atropine makes me beat faster. Now, let's put the pedal to the metal!

Regional anesthetics

Spinal and epidural anesthetics are types of regional anesthesia that anesthetize a specific body region while the patient remains conscious.

Spinal anesthesia

In spinal anesthesia, a local anesthetic is injected into the intrathecal (subarachnoid) space, puncturing the dura and blocking sensation in the lower body.

The local anesthetic blocks nerve impulse transmission, inhibiting both sensory and motor sensation. Typically, the anesthesiologist injects the drug at the third or fourth lumbar space, using a 26G or other small, hollow needle.

Spinal anesthetics	Indications	Adverse reactions	Nursing considerations
■ procaine ■ tetracaine ■ bupivicaine ■ lidocaine	Spinal anesthetics are used to block sensation in the lower body for surgery.	■ Hypotension ■ Respiratory paralysis ■ Hematoma ■ Infection at the injection site ■ Postlumbar puncture (post-spinal) headache	■ Monitor blood pressure, heart rate, oxygen saturation, urine output, and pain relief. ■ Position your patient with the head of the bed at 0 to 30 degrees to avoid postspinal headache.

Patient positioning for spinal anesthesia

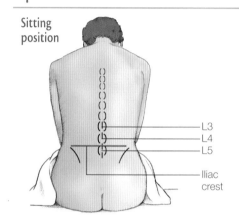

Sitting position

L3
L4
L5

Iliac crest

Epidural anesthesia

In epidural anesthesia (also called an *epidural block*), a local anesthetic, an opioid, or both is injected into the epidural space outside the spinal canal without puncturing the dura. The intravertebral space used depends on the location of the surgical procedure.

The anesthetic causes local sensation loss. With epidural anesthesia, a 17G or 18G blunt-tipped needle is used to inject the drug.

Epidural anesthetics	Indications	Adverse reactions	Nursing considerations
■ chloroprocaine ■ lidocaine ■ bupivacaine	■ Epidural anesthetics are used to block sensation for surgery and to reduce pain in women in labor.	■ Hypotension ■ Fever ■ Pruritus ■ Urinary retention ■ Respiratory depression ■ Hematoma ■ Infection at injection site ■ Paresthesia	■ Monitor blood pressure, oxygen saturation, urine output, and pain relief. ■ The risk of postspinal headache with epidural anesthesia is rare (occurs with unintentional dura puncture).

Local anesthetics

Local anesthetics prevent or relieve pain in a specific body area. They're commonly given with spinal or epidural anesthesia or with a peripheral nerve block as an alternative to general anesthesia.

Local anesthetics work by blocking nerve impulses. As they accumulate, the cell membrane expands and the cell becomes unable to depolarize. This blocks pain impulse transmission.

Local anesthetics fall into two classes — amides and esters.

Lateral position

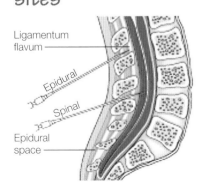

Epidural and spinal anesthesia injection sites

Ligamentum flavum

Epidural

Spinal

Epidural space

Local anesthetics	Indications	Adverse reactions	Nursing considerations
Amides *Long-acting* ■ bupivacaine hydrochloride (Marcaine) ■ ropivacaine hydrochloride (Naropin) *Intermediate-acting* ■ lidocaine hydrochloride (Xylocaine) ■ mepivacaine hydrochloride (Carbocaine) ■ prilocaine hydrochloride (Citanest) **Esters** *Long-acting* ■ tetracaine hydrochloride (Pontocaine) *Short-acting* ■ chloroprocaine hydrochloride (Nesacaine) ■ procaine hydrochloride (Novocain)	■ Local anesthetics are used to block pain in a specific body area. ■ They're also used as an alternative to general anesthesia.	■ Anxiety ■ Apprehension ■ Restlessness ■ Nervousness ■ Disorientation ■ Confusion ■ Dizziness ■ Blurred vision ■ Tremors ■ Twitching ■ Shivering ■ Seizures ■ Myocardial depression ■ Bradycardia ■ Arrhythmias ■ Hypotension ■ Cardiovascular collapse ■ Cardiac arrest	■ Assess for signs and symptoms of local anesthetic toxicity. ■ Know which local anesthetic the patient received and which technique (such as spinal, epidural, or peripheral nerve block) was used. ■ Local anesthetics that contain vasoconstrictors, such as epinephrine, can cause both CNS and cardiovascular reactions.

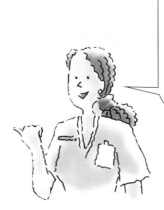

Remember, local anesthetics are divided into two categories — amides and esters — and can be long-, intermediate-, or short-acting.

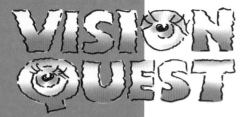

Matchmaker

Match each type of pupil with the anesthesia stage in which it occurs.

1. Stage I _____ A.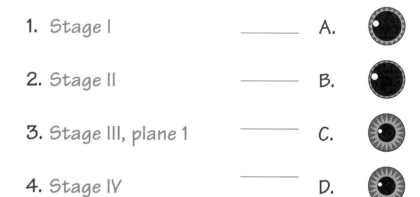

2. Stage II _____ B.

3. Stage III, plane 1 _____ C.

4. Stage IV _____ D.

Able to label?

Identify the sections of the spine and the injection sites for epidural and spinal anesthesia indicated on this illustration.

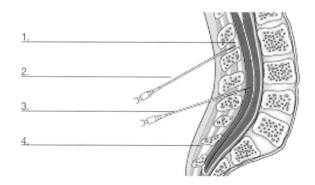

1. _____

2. _____

3. _____

4. _____

3

Perioperative care

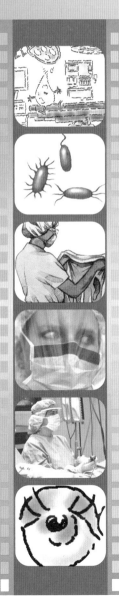

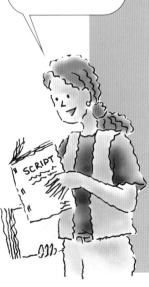

Proper perioperative care ensures that your patient's surgery goes as scripted. Read on to acquaint yourself with your role, and don't forget to rehearse your lines.

SCRIPT

■ Surgical suite environment 40

■ Infection control principles 43

■ Surgical asepsis 46

■ Setting up for OR cases 53

■ Patient arrival in the surgical suite 55

■ Cleanup 61

■ Vision quest 62

Surgical suite environment

> Some surgical suites also contain a pathology laboratory and satellite pharmacy.

Perioperative care involves caring for patients who are undergoing surgical or other invasive procedures.

Surgery may be performed in:
■ traditional hospital-based operating rooms
■ ambulatory surgical centers
■ laser centers
■ mobile surgical units.

Areas within the surgical suite

Although most suites have the same areas, the layout may vary based on the type and size of the unit. Surgical suites commonly contain these areas:
■ operating rooms (ORs) or procedure rooms
■ storage and supply areas (sterile and nonsterile)
■ support areas, including the preoperative holding area or admission area, postanesthesia care unit (PACU) and, occasionally, the anesthesia office.

Design of the surgical suite

The surgical suite is designed to:
■ keep the unit self-contained
■ restrict unauthorized entry
■ centralize personnel, equipment, and supplies
■ control the environment and prevent cross-contamination from other parts of the facility.

The design of the surgical suite may follow one of four basic plans.

> Corridors are designed to control the traffic patterns of personnel, patients, and equipment.

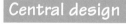

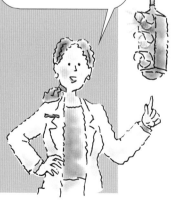

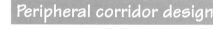

Central design
■ Used for small units with a maximum of 4 ORs
■ Has a single corridor

Peripheral corridor design
■ Used for large units
■ Has a main outer corridor (or outer core) area, plus an inner corridor (or inner core) area

Double-corridor design
■ Used for units with 5 to 15 ORs
■ Has a U- or T-shaped floor plan

Modular design
■ Cluster or pod of ORs designed around a central area

Peripheral corridor design

This floor plan shows a surgical suite in the peripheral corridor design, with both an inner and an outer core.

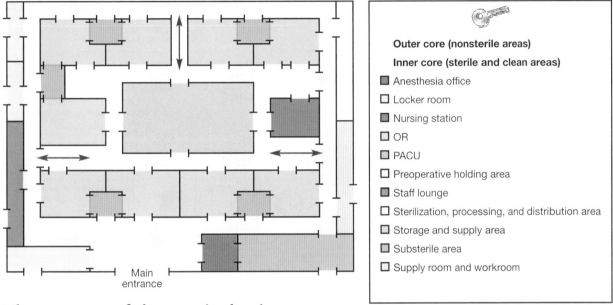

Outer core (nonsterile areas)

Inner core (sterile and clean areas)

- ▤ Anesthesia office
- ☐ Locker room
- ▤ Nursing station
- ☐ OR
- ▥ PACU
- ☐ Preoperative holding area
- ▪ Staff lounge
- ☐ Sterilization, processing, and distribution area
- ▥ Storage and supply area
- ▥ Substerile area
- ☐ Supply room and workroom

Main entrance

Three zones of the surgical suite

No matter how a surgical suite is designed, it's typically divided into three zones to help control the environment and prevent contamination. Each zone is restricted to certain personnel and has its own dress code, supplies, and activities. (These may vary among facilities. See your facility's policy and procedure manual for details.)

Unrestricted zone

Areas
- ▪ Main entrance to surgical suite (where staff, patients, equipment, and supplies enter)
- ▪ Preoperative holding area
- ▪ Admission area
- ▪ PACU
- ▪ Anesthesia office
- ▪ Staff lounge and locker rooms

Clothing required
- ▪ Nursing scrubs and street clothes may be worn.

Semirestricted zone

Areas
- ▪ Peripheral support areas
- ▪ Corridors leading to ORs
- ▪ Storage and supply areas
- ▪ Workroom
- ▪ Sterilization and processing areas

Clothing required
- ▪ Proper OR attire (including surgical scrubs, cap, and shoe covers) is required.
- ▪ All head and facial hair must be covered.

Restricted zone

Areas
- ▪ ORs
- ▪ Substerile areas connected to the ORs (which typically house the scrub sinks, autoclave, and blanket warmer)

Clothing required
- ▪ Proper OR attire (including surgical scrubs, cap, and shoe covers) is required.
- ▪ All head and facial hair must be covered.
- ▪ Masks must be worn when the sterile field is set up for surgery, sterile supplies are open, and surgery is being performed.

Environmental factors in the OR

Air exchange and ventilation system

To prevent airborne contamination, every OR should have an adequate air exchange and filtration system and a positive-pressure ventilation system. The anesthesia machine must have a gas-scavenging system to prevent staff exposure to anesthetic vapors. The OR must also have a smoke evacuation system to prevent staff exposure to smoke plume from lasers and electrosurgical devices.

We need to be kept under control!

Communication system

Each OR must have an effective communication system, including an intercom and a telephone system with access to an outside line. It must also have an emergency alert system to contact additional personnel when needed to assist in an emergency.

Electrical safety

All electrical equipment in the OR must be inspected routinely and meet safety codes to prevent electrical hazards, such as fire, burns, and electric shock. In addition, safety guidelines for specialized equipment, such as lasers, must be followed.

Temperature and humidity control

Temperature and humidity control help prevent the growth of pathogenic organisms. The OR temperature should be maintained between 68° and 73° F (20° to 22.8° C), with a humidity level between 30% and 60%.

Size

The standard OR is a 360-square-foot rectangle or square, with ceiling-mounted lights and fixed cabinets and shelves for emergency equipment and supplies. Larger ORs, of 600 square feet or more, are used for procedures requiring additional equipment, such as open-heart or orthopedic surgery.

Infection control principles

The four main types of microorganisms that cause human infections are bacteria, fungi, parasites, and viruses.

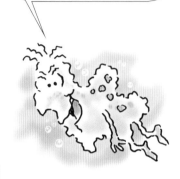

Infection is an invasion and multiplication of microorganisms in or around the body that produces an immune response. Bacteria, including staphylococcus, streptococcus, enterococcus, and pseudomonad, cause most postoperative surgical infections.

Comparing bacterial shapes

Bacteria exist in three basic shapes: rods (bacilli), spheres (cocci), and spirals (spirilla).

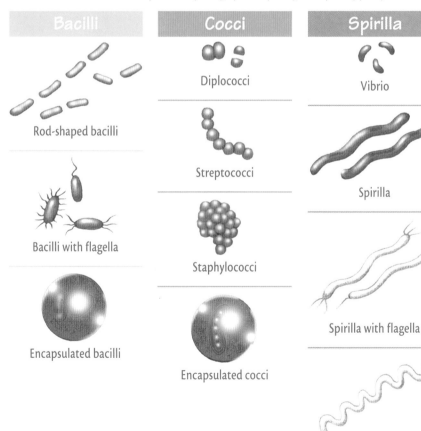

Bacilli	Cocci	Spirilla

Rod-shaped bacilli

Bacilli with flagella

Encapsulated bacilli

Diplococci

Streptococci

Staphylococci

Encapsulated cocci

Vibrio

Spirilla

Spirilla with flagella

Spirochete

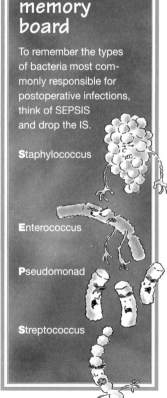

memory board

To remember the types of bacteria most commonly responsible for postoperative infections, think of SEPSIS and drop the IS.

Staphylococcus

Enterococcus

Pseudomonad

Streptococcus

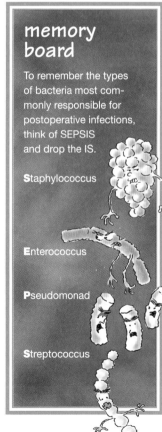

Chain of infection

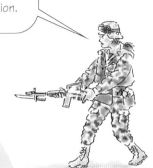

An infection can occur only if all six components shown here are present. Removing one link in the chain prevents infection.

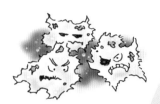

Causative agent

A *causative agent* for infection is any microbe that can produce disease.

Susceptible host

Transmission of infection requires a *susceptible host*. The human body has many defense mechanisms to keep pathogens from entering and multiplying. When these mechanisms function normally, infection doesn't occur. In a weakened host, an infectious agent is more likely to invade the body and launch infection.

Reservoir

The *reservoir* is the environment or object in or on which a microbe survives and, in some cases, multiplies. Inanimate objects, human beings, and other animals can serve as reservoirs, providing essential requirements for the microbe to survive at specific stages in its life cycle.

Portal of entry

The *portal of entry* is the path by which an infectious agent invades a susceptible host. It's usually the same as the portal of exit.

Portal of exit

The *portal of exit* is the path by which an infectious agent leaves its reservoir. Usually, it's the site where the organism grows. In human reservoirs, common exit portals include the respiratory, GI, and GU tracts; skin and mucous membranes; and placenta (in transplacental disease transmission from mother to fetus). Bodily secretions, such as blood, sputum, and emesis, can also serve as exit portals.

Mode of transmission

The *mode of transmission* is the means by which the infectious agent passes from the portal of exit in the reservoir to the susceptible host. The five modes of transmission are contact, airborne, droplet, common vehicle, and vector-borne. The transmission mode varies with the specific microbe. Some organisms use more than one mode.

Surgical wound classification

The Centers for Disease Control and Prevention has developed a system for classifying surgical wounds based on potential risk factors for postoperative infection. A surgical wound may be clean, clean-contaminated, contaminated, or dirty (infected).

Clean wound

■ Uninfected surgical wound without inflammation in which the respiratory, GI, or GU tract hasn't been entered
■ Examples: surgical wounds from total knee replacement and breast biopsy

Clean-contaminated wound

■ Surgical wound with no sign of infection in which the respiratory, GI, or GU tract has been entered
■ Examples: surgical wounds associated with thoracotomy and abdominal hysterectomy

Contaminated wound

■ Open, fresh traumatic wound or surgical wound involving spillage from the GI tract that may be caused by surgery in which a violation of surgical asepsis has occurred
■ Examples: open fractures and wounds associated with surgery to remove a ruptured appendix

Dirty wound

■ Infected wound, perforated viscera, or old traumatic wound with retained devitalized tissue
■ Examples: wounds caused by debridement or incision and drainage of an abscess

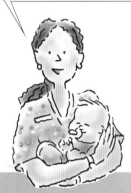

The very young and the very old are at increased risk for postoperative wound infection.

Risk factors for surgical wound infection

■ Age extremes
■ Chronic corticosteroid use
■ Diabetes mellitus
■ Immunosuppression
■ Malnutrition
■ Multiple preoperative coexisting medical disorders
■ Obesity
■ Recent surgery
■ Radiation therapy previously applied to the surgical site
■ Skin-prep hair removal with a razor
■ Wound drains at the surgical site

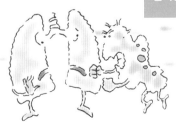

Surgical asepsis

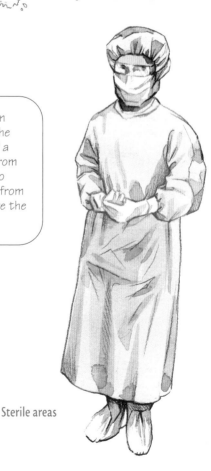

Prepare to die, nasty microbes! We use sterile technique here, so you won't get past the OR door!

Asepsis means the absence of infectious microorganisms. Surgical asepsis—the absence of all microorganisms—is used in the OR to create and maintain a sterile environment, which helps protect the patient from infection.

Principles of asepsis

The OR staff adheres to the following principles during a surgical procedure:
- All items used within the sterile field must be sterile.
- Sterile persons may touch only sterile items or areas of the field. Unsterile persons may touch only unsterile items or areas of the field.
- Movement within or around the sterile field must not contaminate the field.
- Sterile gowns are considered sterile in the front, from the shoulder to the tabletop level of the sterile field, and at the sleeves, from the cuff to 2″ above the elbow.
- Tables are sterile only at tabletop level.
- Edges of a sterile container are considered unsterile once the container has been opened.
- A sterile barrier that has been permeated is considered unsterile.
- Consider all items or areas of doubtful sterility to be contaminated and unsterile.

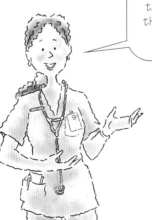

Here you see an illustration of the sterile areas of a sterile gown — from the shoulder to tabletop level and from the cuff to 2″ above the elbow.

Sterile areas

Surgical hand scrub

The surgical hand scrub is crucial to surgical asepsis. Staff members who scrub should be in good health, with intact skin free from cuts and abrasions. Keep nails short and unpolished, and don't wear artificial nails. Before scrubbing, remove all rings, watches, and bracelets.

For the traditional scrub procedure, you'll use individually packaged, disposable surgical sponges and brushes with an antimicrobial agent and a plastic nail cleaner. The sponge is preferred over the brush for scrubbing because it's less traumatic to the skin, especially with repeated scrubbing.

The traditional scrub is timed for 5 minutes, with 2½ minutes for each hand and arm. Some facilities allow 5 minutes for the initial scrub and 3 minutes for subsequent scrubs.

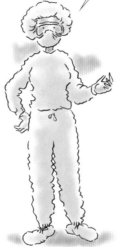

To enter the scrub sink area, your head and facial hair must be completely covered, and you must be wearing a surgical scrub suit, shoe covers, a cap or hood, and a shield mask or goggles.

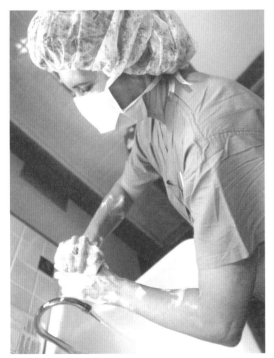

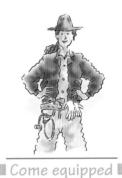

Come equipped

Shield mask

A shield mask like the one shown here protects the wearer's eyes from splashes of blood and other fluids.

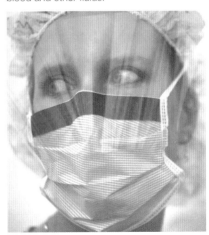

Five-minute surgical scrub

1 Adjust the water temperature to a comfortable level. Wet your hands and forearms, and then lather your hands and arms with soap for prewashing. Follow with a rinse.

2 Remove the scrub sponge from the package and clean under your nails with the plastic nail cleaner.

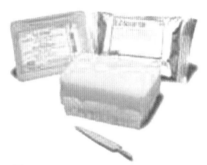

3 Wet the sponge under water to release the antimicrobial soap.

4 Holding the sponge perpendicular to your fingertips, scrub all four sides of each finger, including the finger spaces. Use a back-and-forth motion, and be sure to maintain a good lather throughout.

5 Scrub the palm side and the back of your hand up to the wrist, using a circular motion.

6 Next, scrub all sides of your arm. Start at the wrist and scrub to 2″ above the elbow, rotating your arm from back to front while scrubbing.

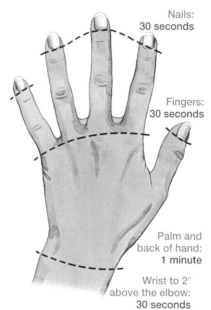

Nails:
30 seconds

Fingers:
30 seconds

Palm and
back of hand:
1 minute

Wrist to 2″
above the elbow:
30 seconds

7 Transfer the sponge to your other hand and repeat steps 4 through 6.

8 Discard the scrub sponge. Rinse your hands and arms from fingertips to elbows. Let excess water drip off your elbows.

9 Enter the OR by backing into the room while holding your hands and arms up in front of your body and keeping your elbows flexed slightly downward. Don't allow your hands or arms to touch your scrub suit.

10 Dry your hands with a sterile towel. (A sterile person must hand you the sterile towel or you can open the package before scrubbing.) Hold the top half of the towel securely in one hand and blot-dry the opposite fingers and hands. Dry your forearm using an upward rotating movement. Next, take the lower end of the towel with your dried hand and repeat the sequence to dry the other hand. (Your hands and arms must be dried with a sterile towel before you put on a sterile gown and gloves in the OR.)

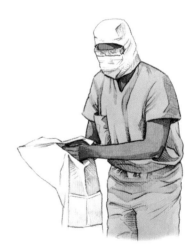

Alcohol-based scrub

Alcohol-based products, which usually combine about 70% alcohol with an antimicrobial and moisturizing agent, are sometimes used as an adjunct to the surgical hand scrub. These products are available as water-aided or waterless types.

The alcohol-based scrub allows for easy application in less time and decreases the use of supplies because a scrub sponge isn't needed. However, you must be aware of the potential fire hazard risk with alcohol products and the need for proper hand-washing technique before using them.

Follow these basic steps when using an alcohol-based scrub product.

■ Wash your hands and forearms with soap and water.

■ Clean your nail beds under running water using a disposable plastic nail cleaner.

■ Thoroughly rinse and dry your hands and forearms.

■ Apply the alcohol-based scrub according to the manufacturer's instructions.

■ Allow your hands to dry completely before putting on sterile gloves. (Alcohol must evaporate completely to reduce the risk of fire hazard.)

Gowning

Sterile surgical staff (surgeon, assistants, and scrub nurse or technician) must wear a sterile gown and gloves. The gown covers the body and scrub suit, helping to maintain the sterile field during surgery. Surgical team members put on surgical gowns with assistance from the circulating nurse.

Putting on a surgical gown

1 Grasp the folded sterile gown at the neckline, using both hands. Step back from the table.

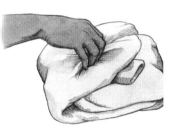

3 Hold the unfolded gown at shoulder level and simultaneously push both hands and arms into the sleeves.

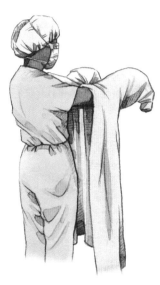

2 Holding the folded gown at the neckline with the inside toward you, keep your hands on the inside of the gown as you let the gown unfold in front of you at arm's length.

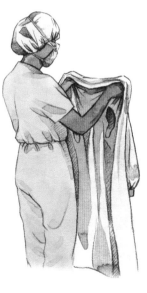

> When putting on a sterile gown, your hands shouldn't extend beyond the gown's cuffs.

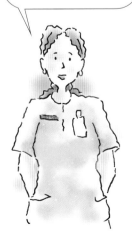

4 The circulating nurse assists by reaching inside the gown to bring the gown over your shoulders. Then she closes and secures the snaps at the neckline and waist.

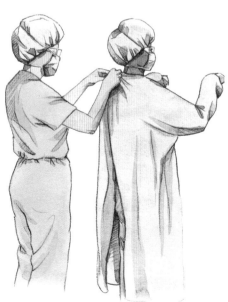

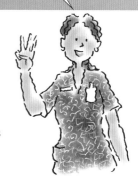

Aren't you lucky? You have three gloving techniques to choose from.

Gloving

Sterile, powder-free surgical gloves serve as a barrier between the patient and staff member, preventing exposure to microorganisms and reducing the risk of surgical site infection. Use sterile, powder-free, nonlatex gloves for staff members and patients with latex sensitivity.

Three gloving techniques exist:
- closed — preferred when initially putting on a sterile gown and gloves
- open — used when sterile gloves are replaced or a sterile gown isn't required
- assisted — used when one team member wearing a sterile gown and gloves helps another team member put on his sterile gloves.

Closed-gloving technique

1 Using the cuff of your gown, open the inside sterile wrapper of the glove package. Lift the first glove off the wrapper by the cuff. Then extend your forearm with the palm upward. Place the glove palm-side down along the forearm of the matching hand, with thumb and fingers pointing toward the elbow. The glove cuff should be over the gown cuff.

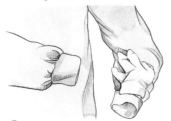

2 Securely hold the glove cuff of the hand being gloved. With the other gown-protected hand, stretch the glove cuff over the end of the gown sleeve and hand.

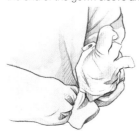

3 Pull the glove on over your extended fingers until it completely covers the gown cuff. Adjust your hand and fingers in the glove.

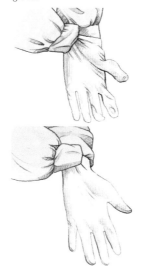

4 Using your gloved hand, pick up the second glove from the sterile wrapper.

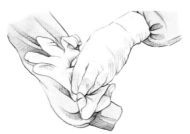

5 Repeat the above procedure with the other hand to put on the second glove.

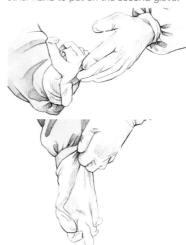

6 Pull the second glove over your extended fingers until it completely covers the gown cuff. Adjust your hand and fingers in the glove.

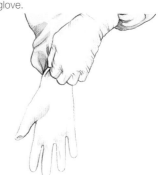

Open-gloving technique

1 Open the glove package by grasping both center folds of the sterile wrapper and spreading the folds apart. Lift the right glove from the wrapper by the edge of the everted glove cuff, using your left thumb and index finger.

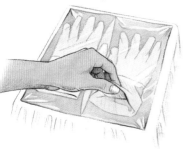

2 Slide the glove over your right hand, holding the glove cuff. Adjust your hand and fingers inside the glove.

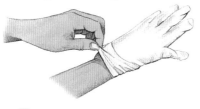

3 Using your gloved right hand, pick up the second glove by placing your gloved fingers under the everted glove cuff. Slide your ungloved left hand into the glove.

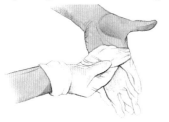

4 Adjust your left hand and fingers in the glove.

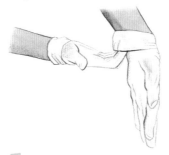

5 Adjust both gloves to cover your wrists (or sterile gown cuff if you're wearing a gown and your gloves are replaced during surgery). Remember, to adjust the gloves, place your gloved fingers under the everted glove cuff and pull the glove upward.

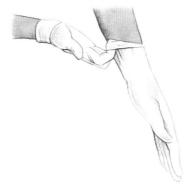

Assisted-gloving technique

1 Wearing a sterile gown and gloves, pick up the right glove from the wrapper by placing your fingers under the everted glove cuff. Hold the glove so its thumb and palm are facing the person you're gloving. Then stretch the glove cuff to allow hand access and maintain sterility.

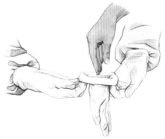

2 Apply resistance as the person you're gloving pushes his hand into the glove.

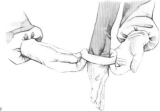

3 Release the glove cuff when the glove is securely in place.

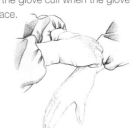

4 Repeat the procedure with the other hand.

Draping

Surgical drapes (disposable sterile drapes and reusable, sterile sheets and towels) are used to create a sterile field. Placed on OR stands and tables, disposable drapes create the sterile surface for holding the sterile instruments, supplies, and other equipment required for surgery.

Usually, the circulating nurse and scrub nurse (or technician) are responsible for placing surgical drapes. Check your facility's policy and procedure manual to be sure.

Keep drapes folded until the time of use. Once you position a drape, it can't be repositioned or allowed to touch the floor.

A sterile team member (scrub nurse or technician) should open a sterile pack from near side to far side. An unsterile team member (such as the circulating nurse) should open a sterile pack from far side to near side. Remember, an unsterile team member must never reach over a sterile field.

Here you see the circulating nurse opening the cover of a pack of sterile drapes. She keeps her fingers under the cover to avoid contact with the sterile parts.

Circulating nurse opening a sterile pack

The surgical conscience at work: As this scrub technician places the sterile drape cover on an OR stand, he keeps his fingers under the drape's cuff to protect his sterile-gloved hands and avoid contamination.

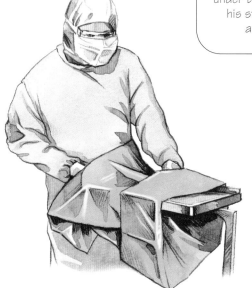

Scrub technician placing a sterile drape cover

Setting up for OR cases

The surgical team refers to the surgeon's preference card when setting up for a surgical procedure. This card lists all the standard instruments, supplies, and equipment needed for the procedure, plus specific items requested by the surgeon.

Surgeon's preference card	
Surgeon name:	Adleri, James, MD
Procedure:	Pacemaker insertion, permanent
Glove size:	7½ Tridil (right-handed)
Patient position:	Supine
Drapes:	Breast hernia pack
	Towels/clips
	(surgeon usually places generator in right chest)
	c – arm drape
Medications:	Lidocaine 1% 50 ml
Skin prep:	E-Z prep
Sutures and needles:	3 – 0 Vicryl 27"
	4 – 0 Vicryl 18"
	3 – 0 Silk 18"
	2 – 0 Prolene
	30G needles
Instruments and trays:	Pacemaker tray
	General forceps DeBakey 7"
Supplies:	Syringe 10-cc
	1,000 ml sterile NSS solution
	100 ml sterile water solution
	Introducer set subclavian 10.0
	Triple-lumen kit
Equipment:	Emergency cart
	c – arm
	Lead aprons — 4
Dressings:	
Notes:	Notify pacemaker representative
	External pacemaker leads
	Generator
Comments:	Pacemaker rep notified by _____

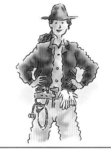

Come equipped

Common surgical instruments

Curette	
Forceps	
Hemostat	
Retractor	
Sound	
Scalpel	

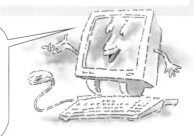

If the surgeon's preference list is computerized, your facility may use it for inventory tracking and charging.

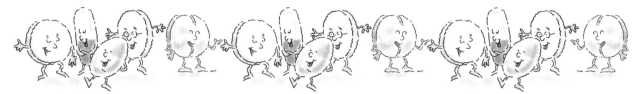

Medication safety

All sterile solutions and medications placed on the sterile field must be labeled.

Components of medication safety in the OR include:
- verifying the medication label
- delivering medications to the sterile field
- using sterile transfer devices
- labeling medications on and off the sterile field (labels used in the sterile field must be sterile)
- confirming labeled medications on the sterile field
- communicating medication strength and dosage to the surgical team member administering it
- establishing dosage limits
- monitoring the patient for adverse drug reactions.

Medication safety is crucial in the OR. Each facility's policy and procedure manual should include a procedure to ensure safe OR medication practices.

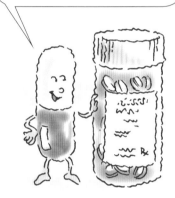

Communication between surgical team members about medications in the OR is always a key component of safety.

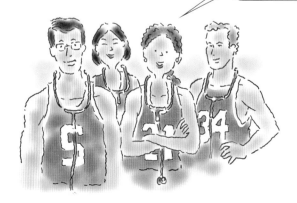

Patient arrival in the surgical suite

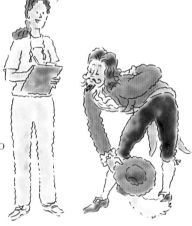

I just need to check your identity. Hmmm...Your date of birth is 1513? Yep — that's what it says on your chart.

While the OR is being prepared for surgery, the patient typically waits in the preoperative holding area. When the patient arrives in the holding area, you must confirm his identity using two patient identifiers. The surgeon may see the patient and obtain consent if he hasn't already done so. You may start the patient's I.V. and, if ordered, perform hair removal. (The night before surgery, the patient usually showers or bathes with an antimicrobial soap.)

Before hair removal, you must verify the correct surgical site. Ideally, you should remove the patient's hair in the OR as close to the time of surgery as possible. To remove hair, use a depilatory (after a patch test to check for skin reactions) or clip it with disposable clippers. Don't use a razor, which may cause skin trauma and increase infection risk.

Hair removal sites

Forearm, elbow, and hand

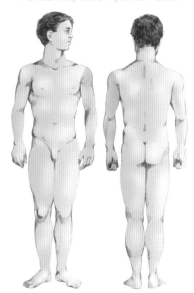

On the operative side, remove hair from the fingertips to the shoulder. Include the axilla, unless surgery is for the hand. Clean and trim the fingernails.

Knee and lower leg

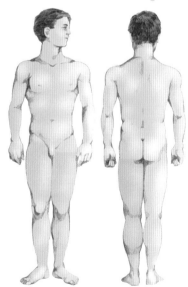

On the operative side, remove hair from the toes to the groin. Clean and trim the toenails.

Abdomen

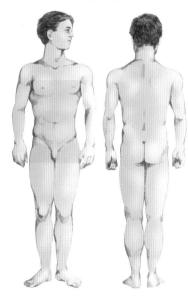

Remove hair from 3″ above the nipples to the upper thighs, including the pubic area.

Patient arrival in the OR

Upon the patient's arrival in the OR, you must confirm his identity again. Then, immediately before starting the procedure, the surgical team stops and takes a "time out" to verify the correct patient, correct procedure, correct surgical site and, if applicable, any surgical implants required. You must document the "time out" on the perioperative flow sheet.

Also document the intraoperative nursing assessment and nursing diagnoses on the perioperative flow sheet.

Key nursing diagnoses for surgical patients

- Acute pain related to the surgical procedure
- Anxiety related to knowledge deficit and stress of surgery
- Hypothermia related to physical, biological, or chemical factors
- Risk for impaired skin integrity related to immobilization, pressure, and shearing forces
- Risk for infection related to invasive procedures
- Risk for injury related to transfer and transport
- Risk for perioperative-positioning injury

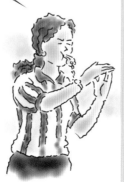

The surgical team's "time-out" is crucial to preventing OR errors and must be documented on the perioperative flow sheet.

Perioperative flow sheet

Patient's full name: _____ Date: _____

Procedure: _____
_____

Suite #:	Procedure start:	Time patient in room:	Anesthesia start:
ASA Score:	Procedure end:	Time patient out of room:	Anesthesia finish:

Anesthesia provider:

Surgeon :	Pathology specimens:
Assistant 1:	Routine: _____
Circulating nurse:	Frozen section: _____
Scrub assistant:	Cultures: _____

Intraoperative nursing data

■ RISK FOR INFECTION

☐ Skin intact pre-op ☐ Other: _____
☐ Surgical clippers: _____
   Area: _____
☐ Skin prep By: _____
   ☐ Povidone iodine ☐ Chlorhexidine ☐ Other _____
Wound classification:
   ☐ Clean ☐ Clean-contaminated ☐ Contaminated ☐ Dirty
☐ Urinary catheter:
   Size/type:_____
   OR output _____ Inserted by: _____
☐ Drains/tubes (size/type/site): _____
   OR drainage amount: _____
☐ Packing (size/type/site): _____
☐ Cast (type/site): _____
☐ Dressing (type/site): _____

■ RISK FOR HYPOTHERMIA
☐ Apply warming blanket #: _____
   Temp setting:_____ Applied by: _____
☐ Warm I.V. fluid
☐ Warm irrigation
☐ Other: _____

Operating room patient identification:

Operative procedure and site: _____

_____

Surgeon	Circ Nurse	
☐	☐	Patient ID bracelet personally observed
☐	☐	Patient questioned verbally regarding ID, Procedure, and Site
☐	☐	Patient's chart reviewed to verify ID, Procedure, and Site
☐	☐	Surgical site confirmed
☐	☐	Time-out performed

Implants/Prosthesis ☐ Yes ☐ No   Exp. Date:_____
  Manufacturer: _____
  Type: _____
  Size: _____
  Lot/Serial #: _____

_____

Surgeon's Signature   Time

_____

Circulating Nurse's Signature   Time

■ RISK FOR IMPAIRED SKIN INTEGRITY

Position for surgery: ☐ Supine ☐ Prone ☐ Lithotomy
                       ☐ L lateral ☐ R lateral ☐ Other:_____
Positioning devices: ☐ Chest roll ☐ Shoulder roll ☐ Axillary roll
                      ☐ Pillow ☐ Stirrups ☐ Leg holder
Pad bony prominences: ☐ Elbows ☐ Heels ☐ Arms tucked
                       Other: _____

■ RISK FOR INJURY
☐ Apply safety strap to: _____
☐ Apply grounding pad Site: _____
☐ Electrosurgical unit #: _____ ☐ Bipolar #:_____
  Setting: Coag: _____ Cut: _____
☐ Laser Type:_____ Unit #:_____ Settings:_____ Time:_____
  ☐ Safety measures implemented Operator:_____
☐ Tourniquet checked & applied #:_____ Site:_____
  Applied by: _____
  ☐ Inflated:_____ ☐ Deflated:_____ Pressure:_____
Sequential stockings: ☐ Yes ☐ No ☐ Other:_____ Unit #: _____

_____

RN's Signature   Time

Perioperative documentation must include:
■ patient's biographical data
■ procedure and surgical team information
■ nursing assessment
■ specimen care and handling
■ count sheet, which documents the number of sponges, sharps, and instruments used during surgery.

Items to include on the count sheet may vary among facilities. See your facility's policy and procedure manual for which items must be counted, the number of times the count must be performed, and other required documentation. In some facilities, the count sheet is included in the perioperative flow sheet.

Instrument count sheet

Patient's full name: _____ Date: _____
Procedure: _____

Instruments	Set count	First count	Add	Final count
Allis				
Criles				
Forceps				
Hemostats				
Kellys				
Knife handles				
Needle holders				
Prep sticks				
Scissors				
Towel clips				

Count verification:
First count correct
  ☐ Yes   ☐ No
Final count correct
  ☐ Yes   ☐ No
If incorrect, X-ray taken
  ☐ Yes   ☐ No

Circulating RN's signature:

_____

The count sheet helps you keep track of equipment used during surgery.

Patient positioning in the OR

Supine or dorsal recumbent position

The patient is placed flat on her back. The most commonly used — and most natural—position, the supine position allows access to the abdominal and thoracic cavities, head, neck, arms, and legs.

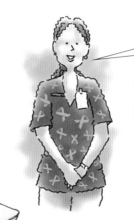

Four positions are commonly used in the OR. Positioning depends on the type of surgery being performed.

Lithotomy position

The patient lies supine with her legs and thighs flexed and supported in stirrups. This position allows access to the perineum and is used for gynecologic, rectal, and urologic procedures.

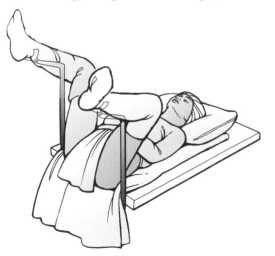

Trendelenburg position

The patient's head and upper body are lowered and her feet are raised. This variation of the supine position allows access to the lower abdomen and pelvis.

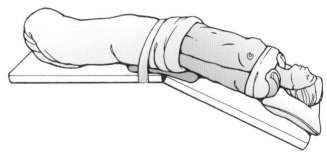

Lateral or Sims' position

The patient lies on the nonoperative side. The lower leg is flexed at the knee and hip, the upper leg is extended, and a pillow is placed between the legs. This position allows access to the upper chest and kidney.

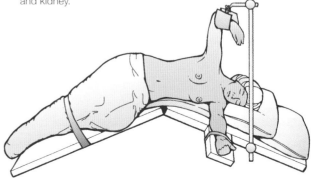

Surgical skin preparation

After the patient is positioned on the OR table, the appropriate team member cleans the skin at and around the expected incision site with an antimicrobial solution. This reduces the number of skin bacteria and the risk of postoperative wound infection. Skin preparation usually takes about 5 minutes.

Wearing sterile gloves, use small circular motions to scrub from the expected incision site to the outer skin periphery, which should be at least 12″ (30.5 cm) from the incision site.

If the incision site is infected, start at the outer border (the cleaner area) and work toward the inner area (the dirty area).

Don't let the antimicrobial solution pool under the patient because this can cause skin irritation.

Remove any drapes used during preparation. Then prepare the patient for surgical draping.

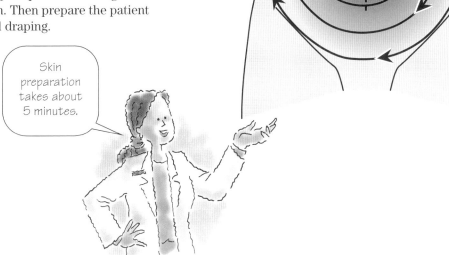

Skin preparation takes about 5 minutes.

Draping the patient for surgery

The patient and OR table are covered with sterile drapes, leaving only the surgical incision site, the arm with the I.V. line, and the patient's head exposed.

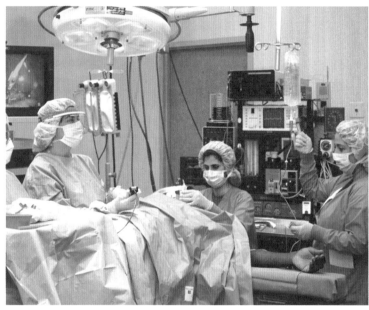

Anesthesiologist at the patient's head

> The surgical patient's head is left exposed so that the airway is accessible to the anesthesiologist, who's responsible for airway maintenance.

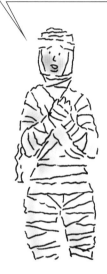

> Sterile drapes, which expose the incision site and isolate it from surrounding areas, are placed to create the sterile field.

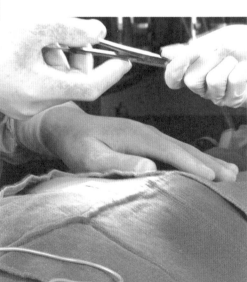

Exposing the incision site

Cleanup

After surgery, the sterile field must be maintained until the patient is ready for transfer to the PACU. Each facility's policy and procedure manual describes the correct procedure for cleaning the OR and for cleaning and sterilizing surgical equipment and instruments.

Reusable surgical supplies are cleaned and then packaged in preparation for sterilization or decontamination. Sterilization methods include steam, chemical, and physical sterilization.

Fiber-optic equipment and other items that can't be sterilized must be disinfected (a process that involves using a chemical agent to destroy infection-producing microorganisms). Appropriate disinfectants for surgical equipment include:

- alcohol
- chlorine compounds
- glutaraldehyde
- phenolics.

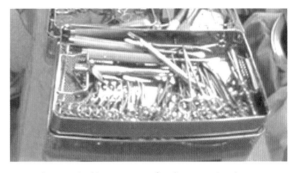

Preparing surgical instruments for decontamination

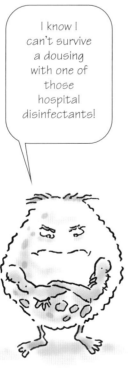

I know I can't survive a dousing with one of those hospital disinfectants!

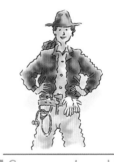

Come equipped

Steam sterilizer

The steam sterilizer heats steam under pressure to a high temperature, which destroys microorganisms on surgical instruments.

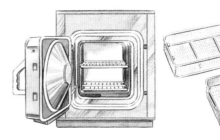

VISION QUEST

Rebus riddle

Sound out each group of pictures and symbols to reveal a principle of asepsis.

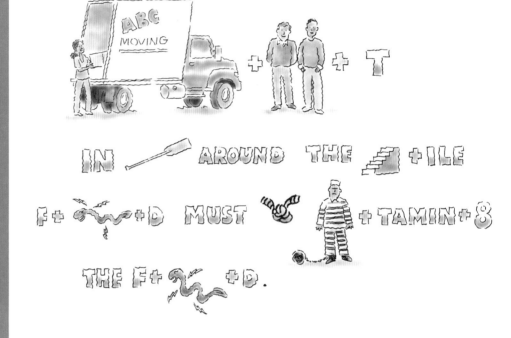

Matchmaker

Match the bacterial shapes with their corresponding names.

1. Cocci _____ A.

2. Bacilli _____ B.

3. Spirilla _____ C.

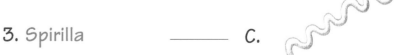

62

4

Procedures

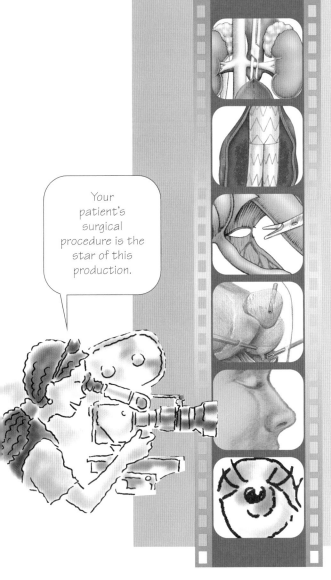

Your patient's surgical procedure is the star of this production.

- Abdominal aortic aneurysm repair to Breast cancer surgery 64

- Carotid endarterectomy to Craniotomy 78

- Femoral bypass grafting to Hysterectomy 90

- Joint replacement to Prostatectomy 102

- Thoracotomy to Valvular surgery 112

- Vision quest 122

Pro

Abdominal aortic aneurysm repair

An abdominal aortic aneurysm (AAA) is an abnormal dilation of the wall of the abdominal aorta. If it ruptures, the patient's life is in danger. To repair an AAA, the surgeon either resects the aneurysm or places an endovascular graft.

AAA resection

During resection, the surgeon removes the aortic segment where the aneurysm is located. He first makes an incision to expose the aneurysm site and clamps the aorta above and below the aneurysm. He then opens the aneurysm sac (usually below the renal arteries). Next, he resects the aneurysm and repairs the damaged segment of the aorta by sewing a prosthetic graft into place.

During anastomoses, the surgeon releases the clamps slowly to test the suture lines and remove clots. After the graft is securely in place and bleeding is controlled, the wound is closed.

Exposing the aneurysm

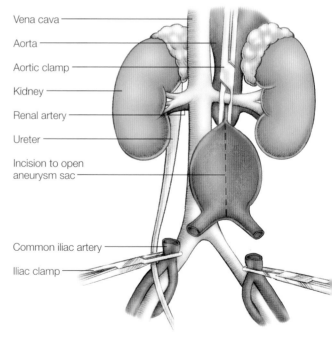

- Vena cava
- Aorta
- Aortic clamp
- Kidney
- Renal artery
- Ureter
- Incision to open aneurysm sac
- Common iliac artery
- Iliac clamp

Endovascular grafting

A minimally invasive procedure for repairing an AAA, endovascular grafting reinforces the aorta's walls. This helps prevent the aneurysm from enlarging or rupturing.

To place an endovascular graft, the surgeon uses fluoroscopic guidance to insert a delivery catheter with an attached compressed graft through a small incision into the femoral or iliac artery. He advances this catheter into the aorta, and then positions it across the aneurysm. A balloon on the catheter is used to expand the graft and affix it to the vessel wall.

The procedure usually takes 2 to 3 hours. The patient is instructed to walk the first day after surgery and is discharged in 1 to 3 days.

Endovascular graft for AAA repair

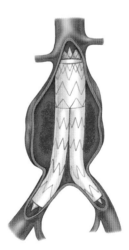

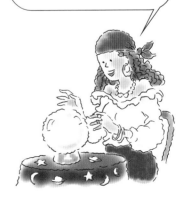

My crystal ball says that a patient who undergoes endovascular grafting will have a shorter hospital stay, smaller abdominal incision, faster return to normal activity, and lower risk of complications.

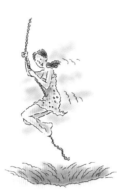

Aortic graft sewn into place

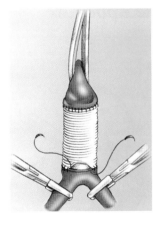

Postop pitfall
Resection risks

Abdominal aortic aneurysm resection may lead to:

■ severe hypotension, from inadequate fluid replacement or sudden blood flow resumption to vessels below the aneurysm
■ renal failure, if problems arise during surgery and clamp time is prolonged.

Be sure to assess your patient's blood pressure frequently. Also, monitor his renal status closely by measuring fluid intake and output and assessing for hematuria.

Appendectomy

With rare exception, appendectomy (appendix removal) is the only effective treatment for acute appendicitis. A common emergency surgery, appendectomy is performed to prevent imminent rupture or perforation of the inflamed appendix. Unless rupture is suspected, most appendectomies are done laparoscopically.

Laparoscopic appendectomy

The surgeon makes three small incisions in the abdomen for trocar placement and the introduction of the laparoscope (with attached video camera) and surgical instruments. He then insuflates the abdominal cavity with carbon dioxide to aid visualization. He uses grasping forceps and stapling instruments to transect the appendix. Then the surgeon cauterizes the appendiceal stump and removes the appendix through the umbilical incision. He irrigates and suctions the abdomen and closes the incisions.

Trocar placement

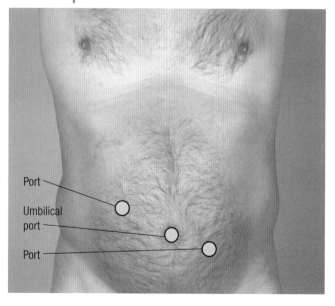

Port

Umbilical port

Port

Transecting the appendix

Stapling device

Cautery

Appendix

Appendectomy

To expose the appendix and isolate it from the bowel attachment, the surgeon makes an incision in the right lower abdominal quadrant, using a transverse or oblique incision over McBurney's point.

   Then he places a purse-string suture in the cecum near the base of the appendix and ligates the base. After cauterizing the appendiceal stump, he ties the purse-string suture securely. He irrigates the wound and removes excess fluid or tissue debris from the abdominal cavity. Finally, he closes the incision.

Laparoscopic appendectomies are the norm, but an open procedure may be performed if rupture is suspected.

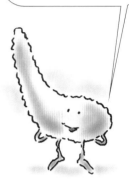

Incision over McBurney's point

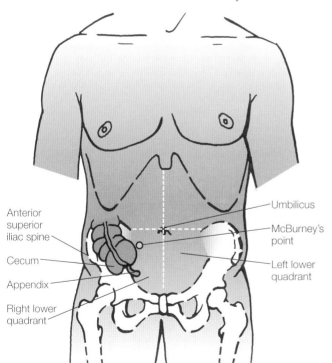

Anterior superior iliac spine

Cecum

Appendix

Right lower quadrant

Umbilicus

McBurney's point

Left lower quadrant

Isolating the appendix

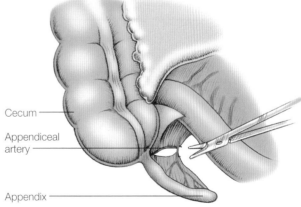

Cecum

Appendiceal artery

Appendix

Arthroscopy

A common endoscopic procedure, arthroscopy is used to directly visualize a joint, allowing the surgeon to assess for problems, plan surgical approaches, document pathology, and diagnose and treat joint disorders. The procedure is most commonly performed on the knee, shoulder, and wrist.

The surgeon inserts the arthroscope into the patient's joint through a puncture. Through two additional punctures, he manipulates additional instruments, such as scissors, shaving knives, and forceps.

Knee arthroscopy

To perform knee arthroscopy, the surgeon inserts a large-bore needle into the suprapatellar pouch and injects sterile saline solution to distend the joint. He passes the arthroscope (with attached video camera) through puncture sites lateral or medial to the tibial plateau. Then he removes articular debris and small, loose bodies.

This procedure may also be done to repair a torn meniscus, reconstruct the anterior cruciate ligament, or take a synovial biopsy or shaving of the patella, cartilage, or meniscus.

Surgeon's view during arthroscopy

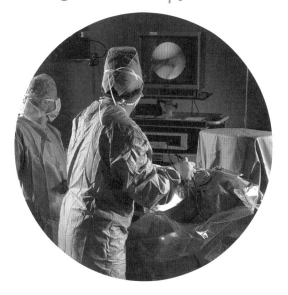

Arthroscope positioned in knee

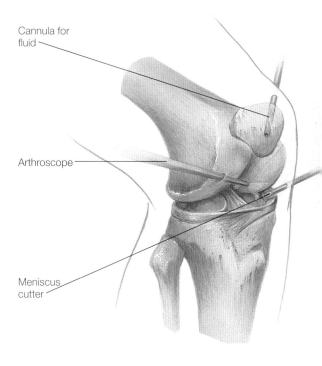

Cannula for fluid

Arthroscope

Meniscus cutter

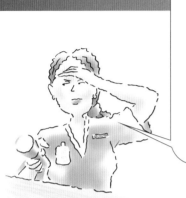

The arthroscope is a fiber-optic instrument with an attached video camera and light source. The camera relays images to video monitors in the operating room, giving the surgical team an inside view.

Shoulder arthroscopy

In shoulder arthroscopy, the surgeon inserts a large-bore needle into the posterior soft spot of the joint capsule and directs it toward the coracoid process. Then sterile saline solution is injected into the glenohumeral joint, and the surgeon passes the arthroscope (with attached video camera) through the puncture site of the posterior joint capsule. While visualizing the shoulder joint, he can remove loose bodies, lyse adhesions, take a synovial biopsy, perform synovectomy, relieve impingement syndrome, or repair biceps tendon and rotator cuff tears.

Exploring the meniscus

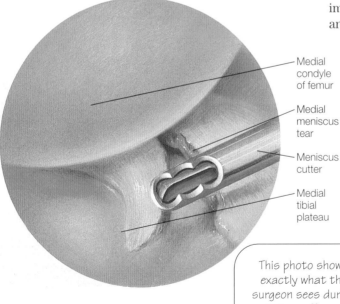

Medial condyle of femur

Medial meniscus tear

Meniscus cutter

Medial tibial plateau

Surgeon's view during rotator cuff repair

This photo shows exactly what the surgeon sees during rotator cuff repair.

Op sight

Bariatric surgery

Bariatric (weight-loss) surgery is performed on the stomach, intestines, or both to promote weight loss in extremely obese patients. After surgery, the patient's food intake is restricted.

Bariatric procedures fall into two main categories:

■ Restrictive procedures limit food intake by reducing the capacity of the stomach without interfering with normal digestion. These procedures include vertical banded gastroplasty and adjustable gastric banding.

■ Combined malabsorptive and restrictive procedures restrict both food intake and the amount of calories and nutrients the body absorbs. These procedures include gastric bypass and biliopancreatic diversion.

Types of bariatric surgery

Vertical banded gastroplasty

In this common procedure, which may be performed by laparoscopy or laparatomy, the surgeon uses both a band and staples to create the reduced stomach pouch.

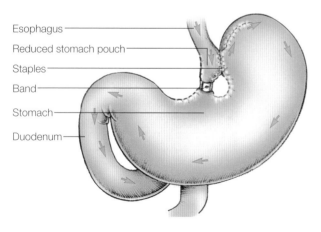

Esophagus
Reduced stomach pouch
Staples
Band
Stomach
Duodenum

Adjustable gastric banding

In this laparoscopic adjustable and reversible procedure, the surgeon places the band around the top of the stomach. The inflation and deflation tube is then inflated 4 weeks postoperatively.

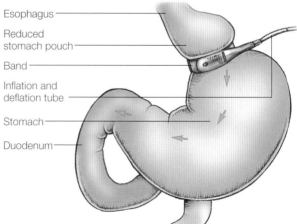

Esophagus
Reduced stomach pouch
Band
Inflation and deflation tube
Stomach
Duodenum

Rarely, a malabsorptive procedure is performed, in which segments of the small intestine are bypassed, reducing the amount of calories absorbed.

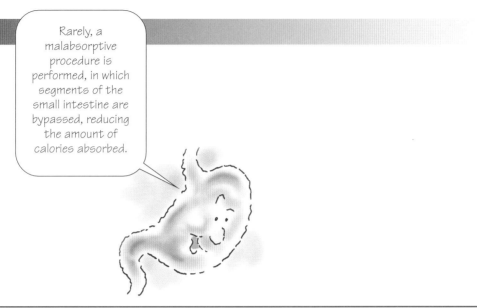

Gastric bypass

In this common procedure, which may be performed by laparoscopy or laparotomy, the surgeon uses sutures and staples with anastomosis to the jejunum to create the reduced stomach pouch.

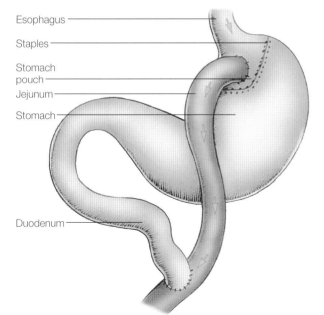

Esophagus

Staples

Stomach pouch

Jejunum

Stomach

Duodenum

Biliopancreatic diversion

In this more complex procedure, the surgeon removes the lower portion of the stomach and anastomoses the remainder of the pouch to the ileum of the small intestines.

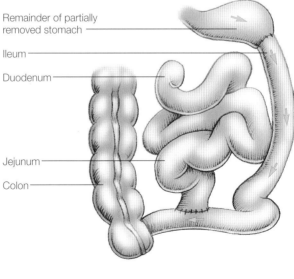

Remainder of partially removed stomach

Ileum

Duodenum

Jejunum

Colon

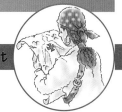

Op sight

Bowel resection

Surgical resection of diseased intestinal tissue and anastomosis (connection) of the remaining segments are used to treat localized obstructive disorders, such as acute diverticulitis, adhesions, and benign or malignant intestinal tumors. Resection is also the preferred treatment for localized bowel cancer.

The surgeon excises diseased colonic tissue and then connects the remaining bowel segments to restore patency. He may use one of two anastomosis techniques:

■ End-to-end anastomosis (ends of two structures are joined) is faster and produces a more physiologically sound junction but requires bowel segments large enough to prevent postoperative obstruction.

■ Side-to-side anastomosis (structures positioned next to each other are joined) reduces the danger of obstruction but takes longer to perform.

Several different types of bowel resection surgery exist, depending on which section of the colon is diseased.

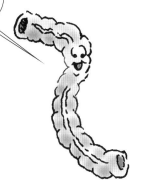

Types of bowel resection

Right hemicolectomy

Indications: Disease of the cecum and lower ascending colon

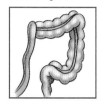

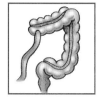

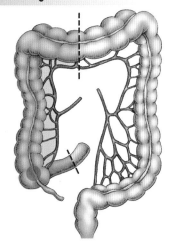

Transverse colectomy

Indications: Disease of the transverse colon

Transverse colon

Descending colon

Ascending colon

Sigmoid colon

Rectum

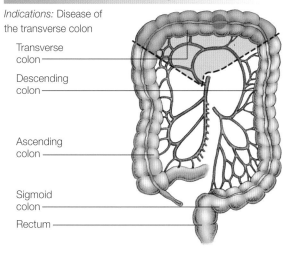

Left hemicolectomy

Indications: Disease of the descending and upper sigmoid colon

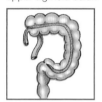

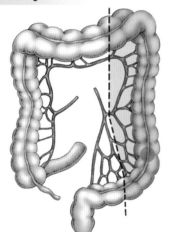

Sigmoid colectomy

Indications: Disease of the lower sigmoid colon or upper rectum

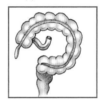

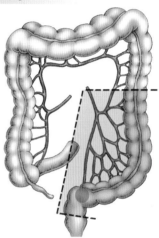

Anterior resection of the sigmoid colon and rectosigmoidostomy

Indications: Disease of the lower sigmoid or rectosigmoid portion of the rectum

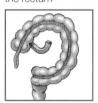

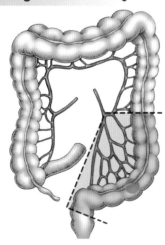

Abdominoperineal resection (Miles' resection)

Indications: Disease of the lower sigmoid colon, rectum, and anus. *Note:* In this procedure, these parts are removed and a permanent colostomy is formed.

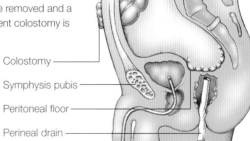

Colostomy

Symphysis pubis

Peritoneal floor

Perineal drain

Urinary catheter

Op sight

Colostomy formation

To resect a large bowel portion because of inflammatory bowel disease, advanced colorectal cancer, or other intestinal maladies, an ostomy may be necessary. In this procedure, the surgeon creates a stoma on the outer abdominal wall to allow feces elimination.

Three stoma construction techniques exist: end, loop, or double barrel.

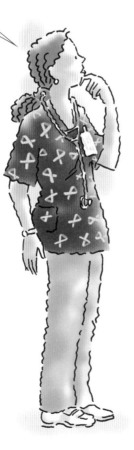

Types of intestinal stomas

End stoma

To form an end stoma, the surgeon pulls a section of the intestine through the outer abdominal wall, everts the section, and sutures it to the skin. An ostomy with an end stoma may be temporary or permanent.

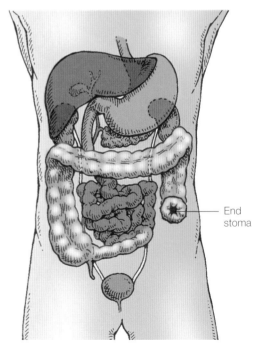

End stoma

Loop stoma

To create a loop stoma, the surgeon brings a loop of intestine out through an abdominal incision to the abdominal surface and supports it with a rod or bridge (usually removed in 5 to 7 days). Then he opens the anterior wall of the bowel loop with a small incision to provide fecal diversion. The result is a stoma with a proximal, functioning limb and a distal, nonfunctioning limb. The surgeon then closes the wound around the exposed intestinal loop.

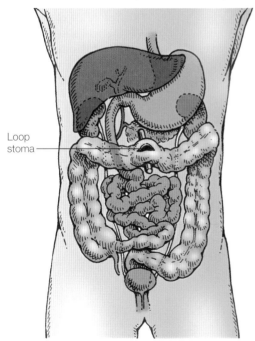

Loop stoma

Double-barrel stoma

For a double-barrel stoma, the surgeon divides the intestine and brings both the proximal and distal ends through the abdominal incision to the abdominal surface. He makes a small incision in the proximal stoma for fecal drainage. The distal stoma (also called a *mucous fistula*) leads to the inactive intestine and is left intact.

Later, when the intestinal injury has healed or the inflammation has subsided, the colostomy is reversed and the divided ends of the intestine are anastomosed to restore intestinal integrity.

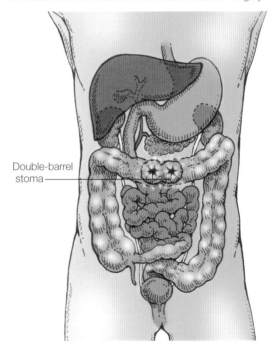

Double-barrel stoma

Breast cancer surgery

Types of surgery for breast cancer include lumpectomy, partial mastectomy, simple (total) mastectomy, modified radical mastectomy, and radical mastectomy. The procedure choice depends on the breast cancer stage and type and the woman's age and menopausal status. Breast reconstruction surgery may also be performed after mastectomy.

In **core needle biopsy,** the surgeon obtains the tissue sample by inserting a cutting-type needle into the breast mass, securing the tissue sample, and withdrawing the needle.

In **sentinel node biopsy,** the surgeon injects dye or radioactive material into the breast mass area in order to identify the sentinel node — the first lymph node along the lymphatic chain of the breast mass. He then removes the node.

In **open breast biopsy,** the surgeon makes an incision over the breast mass and then removes the mass. Open breast biopsy may also be performed with wire localization. (A wire is inserted into the suspicious area before the procedure using the mammogram as a guide.)

Before breast cancer surgery, a breast tissue biopsy and sentinel node biopsy are usually obtained to confirm breast cancer.

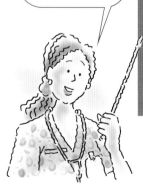

Lumpectomy

Lumpectomy is used to remove small, well-defined lesions. Through a small incision near the nipple, the surgeon removes the breast mass, surrounding tissue and, possibly, nearby axillary lymph nodes. Lumpectomy preserves the breast mound.

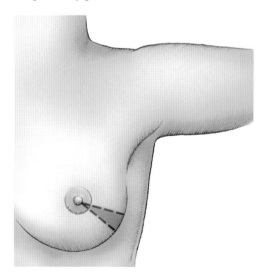

Partial mastectomy

The surgeon makes an incision over the breast mass. Then he removes the breast mass along with enough additional breast tissue to leave tumor-free margins. In some cases, he also removes axillary lymph nodes.

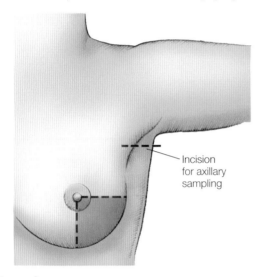

Incision
for axillary
sampling

Simple mastectomy

The surgeon makes an elliptical incision around the breast and then removes the entire breast, leaving axillary lymph nodes and pectoral muscles intact.

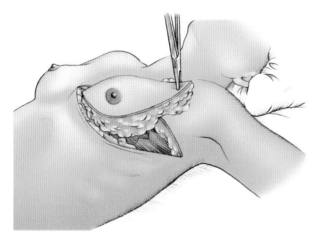

Modified radical mastectomy

Through a transverse or longitudinal incision, the surgeon removes the entire breast, along with some axillary lymph nodes.

Radical mastectomy

The surgeon removes the entire breast, pectoralis major and minor, and axillary lymph nodes. Usually reserved for tumors that have invaded deeper tissues, radical mastectomy has seen declining use in recent years.

Breast reconstruction

Breast reconstruction may be performed either at the time of mastectomy or after a delay. The choice of technique depends on the condition of the patient's skin and underlying tissue. Reconstruction may involve the use of permanent implants, tissue expanders, or myocutaneous flaps.

Two types of flap procedures exist. Both are done in a single stage.

Transverse rectus abdominis myocutaneous

In this most commonly used breast reconstruction procedure, the surgeon tunnels the flap of the rectus abdominis muscle through the abdomen to the mastectomy site. After positioning the flap, he forms the breast mound and sutures the flap in place.

Latissimus dorsi flap

The large, wide latissimus dorsi muscle is used as a flap when a large amount of breast tissue needs to be replaced. The surgeon tunnels the flap under the axilla to the chest wall. After positioning the flap, he places a breast implant (if the patient has insufficient tissue to form a breast mound) and sutures the flap in place.

Op sight

Carotid endarterectomy

Carotid endarterectomy is used to remove atheromatous plaque from the inner lining of the carotid artery. This procedure increases carotid artery blood flow, improving intracranial perfusion. It may be performed with or without a shunt.

To prevent arterial narrowing, the surgeon may place an autogenous saphenous vein patch graft or a synthetic patch.

Endarterectomy with shunt placement

The surgeon makes an incision along the anterior border of the sternocleidomastoid muscle or transversely in a skin crease in the neck. He exposes the common carotid, external carotid, and internal carotid arteries, and then clamps these arteries to evaluate cerebral perfusion. If perfusion is inadequate, he inserts a shunt to permit blood to flow past the obstruction and to ensure adequate cerebral circulation during surgery.

After the artery is stabilized, a heparin infusion is started to prevent thrombosis. The surgeon clamps the external, common, and internal carotid arteries, incises the affected artery, and dissects the plaque.

After plaque removal, the site is flushed to remove debris. Then the shunt is removed and the artery is closed with or without a patch. Clamps are removed sequentially—first from the external carotid, then from the common carotid and, finally, from the internal common carotid artery. The wound is closed and a dressing is applied.

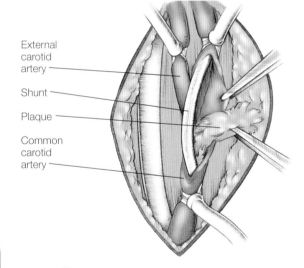

External carotid artery

Shunt

Plaque

Common carotid artery

Make sure to closely monitor your patient's blood pressure and heart rate for the first 24 hours after endarterectomy.

Endarterectomy with synthetic patch graft

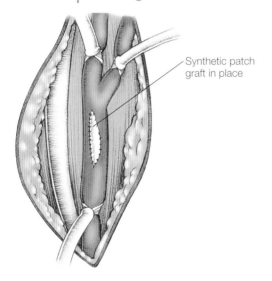

Synthetic patch graft in place

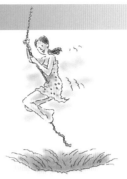

Postop pitfall
Endarterectomy risks

Carotid endarterectomy may cause:
- blood pressure fluctuations
- stroke (if a portion of the plaque embolizes to the brain)
- hyperperfusion syndrome.

For the first 24 hours after the procedure, be sure to monitor your patient's blood pressure and heart rate closely because of surgically induced carotid baroreceptor sensitivity.

Also monitor his cranial nerve function. Cranial nerves VII, X, XI, and XII are situated near the carotid endarterectomy site.

Endarterectomy without shunt placement

If the patient has adequate cerebral perfusion when the carotid arteries are clamped, the surgeon doesn't insert a shunt. Instead, he incises the affected artery and peels plaque away from it. Then he closes the artery with very fine stitches — either directly or with a patch.

Finally, the site is flushed, clamps are removed, the wound is closed, and a dressing is applied.

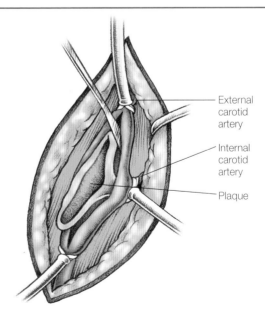

External carotid artery

Internal carotid artery

Plaque

Op sight

Cataract extraction

A common cause of vision loss, a cataract is a gradually developing opacity (clouding) of the lens or lens capsule of the eye. Cataracts commonly affect both eyes, but each cataract progresses independently. They're most common after age 70.

Cataracts can be removed by extracapsular or intracapsular techniques.

Cataract extraction methods

Extracapsular extraction

In extracapsular extraction, the surgeon may use irrigation and aspiration or phacoemulsification. In irrigation and aspiration, he makes an incision at the limbus, opens the anterior lens capsule with a cystotome, and exerts pressure from below to express the lens. Then he irrigates and suctions the remaining lens cortex. In phacoemulsification, the surgeon uses an ultrasonic probe to break up the lens into minute particles. Then he aspirates the particles with the probe.

Irrigation and aspiration

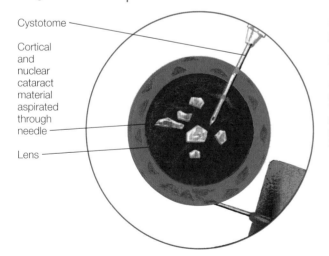

Cystotome

Cortical and nuclear cataract material aspirated through needle

Lens

Phacoemulsification

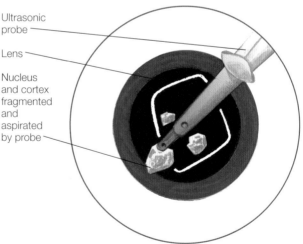

Ultrasonic probe

Lens

Nucleus and cortex fragmented and aspirated by probe

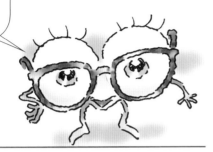

Boy, am I sure glad that cataracts can be removed!

Stages of cataract development

A cataract develops in four stages.

1 **Immature:** The lens isn't totally opaque.

2 **Mature:** The lens is completely opaque, and vision loss is significant.

3 **Tumescent:** The lens is filled with water, and glaucoma may occur.

4 **Hypermature:** Lens proteins deteriorate, causing peptides to leak through the lens capsule. Glaucoma may develop if intraocular fluid outflow is obstructed.

Intracapsular extraction

In intracapsular extraction, the surgeon makes a partial incision at the superior limbus arc. Then he removes the lens using specially designed forceps or a cryoprobe, which freezes and adheres to the lens to aid its removal. This procedure is rarely used today.

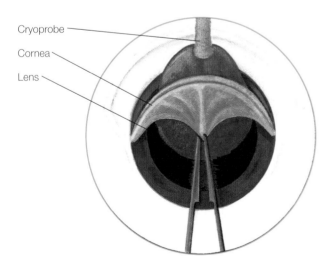

Cryoprobe

Cornea

Lens

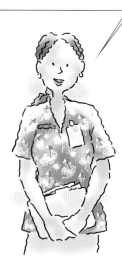

Op sight

Cerebral aneurysm repair

In a cerebral aneurysm, weakness in the wall of a cerebral artery causes localized dilation. Blood flow exerts pressure against that part of the wall, stretching it like a balloon and posing the danger of rupture. Cerebral aneurysms usually arise at the bifurcation in the circle of Willis and its branches.

> A patient is prepared for cerebral aneurysm surgery as soon as his condition stabilizes. The goal of surgery is to reduce the risk of bleeding or rebleeding, vasospasm, and cerebral infarction.

Common cerebral aneurysm sites

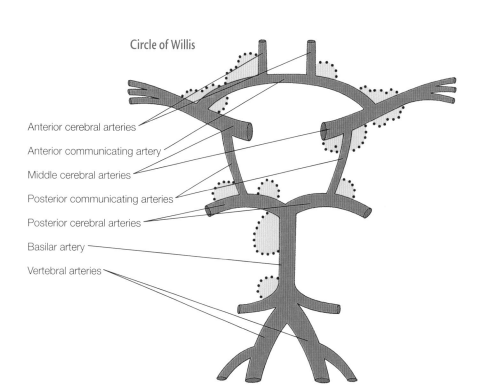

Circle of Willis

Anterior cerebral arteries

Anterior communicating artery

Middle cerebral arteries

Posterior communicating arteries

Posterior cerebral arteries

Basilar artery

Vertebral arteries

Aneurysm repair techniques include clipping and wrapping the aneurysm. First, the surgeon performs a craniotomy, making an incision into the skull to expose underlying structures. When the aneurysm is exposed, he identifies its neck and either excises or clips the aneurysm. Clipping is used to prevent rupture or rebleeding. If the aneurysm can't be clipped, it's wrapped with a gauzelike material to support it.

When surgery isn't appropriate for intracranial aneurysm repair, the patient may undergo electrothrombosis, an endovascular treatment.

Clipping an aneurysm

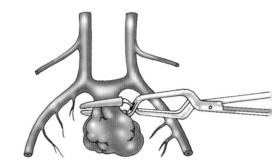

Electrothrombosis for aneurysm repair

Electrothrombosis is most successful for aneurysms with small necks or no significant intrafundal thrombus.

Here's what happens in electrothrombosis:

■ Soft platinum coils soldered to a stainless steel delivery wire are positioned in the fundus of the aneurysm.

■ A 1-mA current is applied to the delivery wire.

■ The delivery wire is removed, leaving the platinum coil in place, and another coil is introduced into the fundus.

■ The process continues until the aneurysm is densely packed with platinum and no longer opacifies during diagnostic contrast injections.

How electrothrombosis works

Theoretically, the positively charged platinum left in the aneurysm attracts negatively charged blood elements, such as white and red blood cells, platelets, and fibrinogen. This causes thrombosis within the aneurysm.

The coils provide immediate protection against further hemorrhage by reducing blood pulsations in the fundus and sealing the hole or weak portion of the artery wall. Eventually, clots form and the aneurysm separates from the parent vessel by formation of new connective tissue.

Platinum is packed into the fundus of the aneurysm to facilitate thrombosis, which causes the aneurysm to separate from the parent vessel.

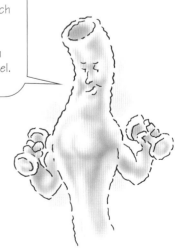

Cholecystectomy

Cholecystectomy (gallbladder removal) is used to treat such disorders as cholecystitis (acute or chronic gallbladder inflammation) and cholelithiasis (gallstones). It's usually performed laparoscopically. When the laparoscopic approach is contraindicated, the open abdominal procedure is used.

Laparoscopic cholecystectomy

The surgeon makes a small incision at the umbilicus for the laparoscope and its attached camera. Then he insufflates the abdomen with carbon dioxide so he can visualize the structures.

   The surgeon makes three more incisions to introduce additional instruments. Then he retracts the gallbladder, exposing the cystic duct. Intraoperative cholangiography may be performed.

   Next, the surgeon clips and divides the cystic duct and dissects the cystic artery and gallbladder. He suctions out bile and any stones and removes the gallbladder through the umbilical port. He may use a specimen bag to secure the gallbladder.

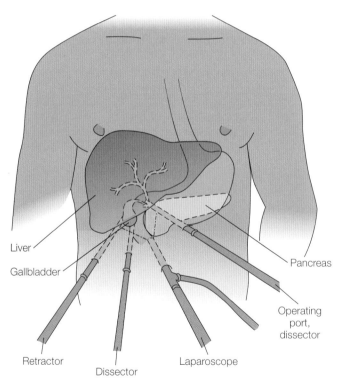

Liver
Gallbladder
Pancreas
Operating port, dissector
Retractor
Dissector
Laparoscope

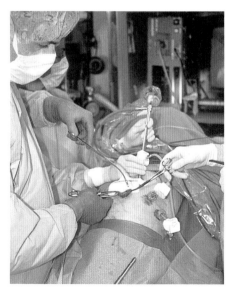

Surgeon performing laparoscopic cholecystectomy

Open abdominal cholecystectomy

Open abdominal cholecystectomy starts with a right subcostal or paramedial incision. The surgeon surveys the abdomen and uses laparotomy packs to isolate the gallbladder from surrounding organs. After identifying biliary tract structures, he may use cholangiography or ultrasonography to help pinpoint the gallstones. With the aid of a choledochoscope, which lets him view the bile ducts directly, he inserts a balloon-tipped catheter to clear stones from the ducts.

Then he ligates and divides the cystic duct and artery and removes the entire gallbladder. He may insert a drain near the cystic duct stump, and then close the wound in layers. Rarely, a T tube is inserted into the common bile duct in the case of retained common bile duct stones.

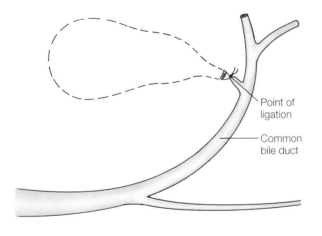

Point of ligation

Common bile duct

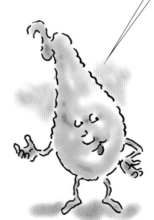

The open abdominal approach is still used to remove the gallbladder if laparoscopy is contraindicated.

Op sight

Coronary artery bypass grafting

In coronary artery bypass grafting (CABG), the surgeon uses an autogenous graft to circumvent an obstruction in a coronary artery caused by buildup of plaque. Conventional CABG surgery is done as an open-heart procedure using cardiopulmonary bypass, which stops the heart temporarily and oxygenates the circulating blood.

A relatively new technique called minimally invasive direct coronary artery bypass (MIDCAB) can be performed on a pumping heart through a small thoracotomy incision.

Understanding cardiopulmonary bypass

In cardiopulmonary bypass, blood is diverted from the heart and lungs to an extracorporeal circuit with minimal hemolysis and trauma. The surgeon inserts catheters into the right atrium or the inferior or superior vena cava for blood removal and into the ascending aorta for blood return.

After heparinizing the patient and priming the pump with fluid to replace diverted venous blood, he switches on the cardiopulmonary bypass ("heart-lung") machine. The pump draws blood from the vena cava catheters into the machine, where blood passes through a filter, an oxygenator, a heat exchanger, and another filter and bubble trap before returning to the arterial circulation. An anesthesiologist or perfusionist maintains mean arterial pressure by adjusting the perfusion rate or infusing fluids or vasopressor drugs.

This heart-lung machine gives me a chance to nap.

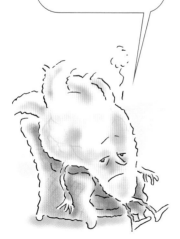

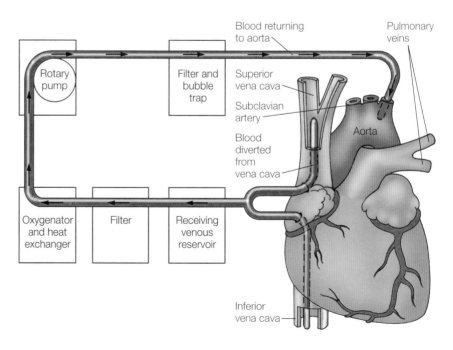

CABG procedure

After the patient receives general anesthesia, CABG surgery begins with graft harvesting. The surgeon makes a series of incisions in the thigh or calf and removes a saphenous vein segment for grafting.

Exposing the heart

Next, the surgeon performs a medial sternotomy to expose the heart. Then he initiates cardiopulmonary bypass. To protect the heart and reduce myocardial oxygen demands during surgery, he induces cardiac hypothermia and standstill by injecting a cold, cardioplegic solution (potassium-enriched saline solution) into the aortic root.

One fine sewing lesson

After the patient is prepared, the surgeon sutures one end of the venous graft to the ascending aorta and the other end to a patent coronary artery distal to the occlusion. To promote proper blood flow, he sutures the graft in a reversed position. He repeats this procedure for each occlusion to be bypassed.

Finishing up

With the grafts in place, the surgeon flushes the cardioplegic solution from the heart; when the heart is contracting gradually, he ends cardiopulmonary bypass. Then he implants epicardial pacing electrodes, inserts a chest tube, closes the incision, and applies a sterile dressing.

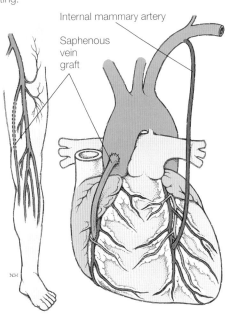

Internal mammary artery

Saphenous vein graft

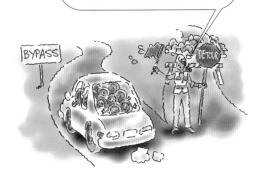

That's right — you all need to follow the detour. Take the bypass route and you should get to where you're going without obstruction.

MIDCAB procedure

With the MIDCAB procedure, the patient typically receives only right lung ventilation, along with drugs to slow the heart rate and reduce movement. Eligible patients include those with proximal left anterior descending lesions and some lesions of the right coronary and circumflex arteries.

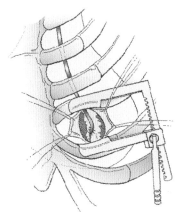

Craniotomy

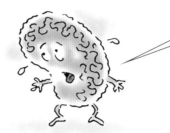

In a craniotomy, the surgeon makes an incision into the skull to expose the brain for such procedures as aneurysm clipping, tumor or abscess excision, hematoma aspiration, or ventricular shunting.

> I need a craniotomy like I need a hole in the head! Come to think of it, a craniotomy IS a hole in the head...

A window to the brain

Initial incision

To perform a craniotomy, the surgeon incises the skin, clamps the aponeurotic layer, and retracts the skin flap. Then he incises and retracts the muscle layer and scrapes the periosteum off the skull.

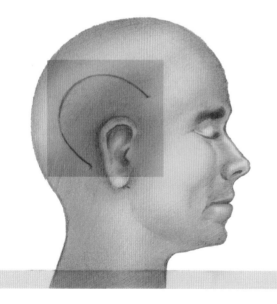

Burr holes drilled

Using an air-driven or electric drill, the surgeon drills a series of burr holes in the corners of the skull incision. During drilling, warm saline solution is dripped into the burr holes, and the holes are suctioned to remove bone dust. If the patient has a subdural hematoma, one burr hole is drilled, the hematoma is evacuated, and a drain is inserted. For hydrocephalus, a ventricular drain is inserted through the burr hole.

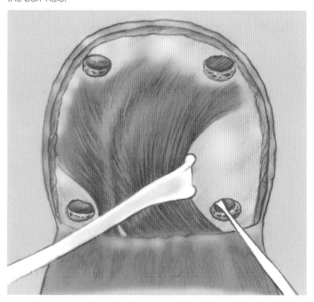

Bone flap removed

For a more complex lesion, such as a tumor or an aneurysm, the surgeon uses a dural elevator to separate the dura from the bone around the margin of each burr hole. Then he saws between burr holes to create a bone flap. He either leaves this flap attached to the muscle and retracts it or detaches the flap completely and removes it. In either case, the flap is wrapped to keep it moist and protected.

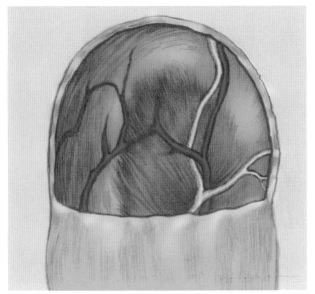

Brain exposed

Finally, the surgeon incises and retracts the dura, exposing the brain.

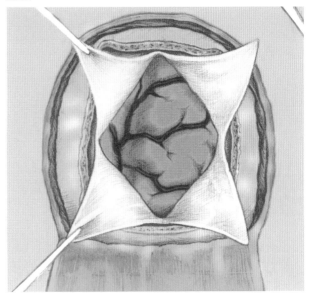

Op sight

Femoral bypass grafting

Bypass grafting is used to reroute blood flow around an obstruction in an artery supplying blood to the leg and foot. After exposing the affected artery, the surgeon anastomoses a synthetic graft to divert blood flow around the occluded segment. The autogenous graft may be a vein or an artery harvested from elsewhere in the patient's body.

Femoropopliteal bypass

A femoropopliteal bypass graft is used to restore blood flow to the leg with a femoral occlusion. The surgeon bypasses the occluded part of the artery with an autogenous graft from the patient's saphenous vein. If this vein can't be used, a synthetic graft is placed.

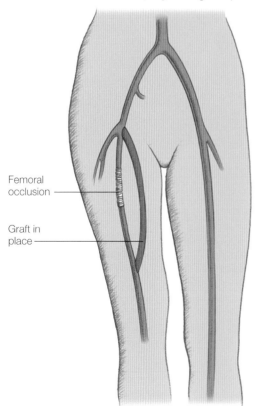

Femoral occlusion

Graft in place

Femorofemoral bypass

A femorofemoral bypass graft, which is outside the normal blood flow pathway, is used to restore blood flow to the leg with an occluded iliac artery. Eligible patients must have good blood flow in the other iliac artery.

The surgeon creates a graft tunnel between the femoral arteries, positions the synthetic graft, and anastomoses it to each femoral artery.

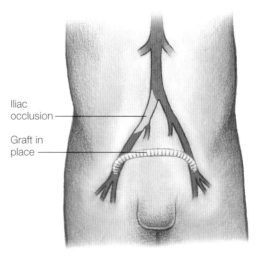

Iliac occlusion

Graft in place

Axillofemoral bypass

An axillofemoral bypass graft is used to restore blood flow to one or both legs in patients with occlusions of one or both iliac arteries. Like the femorofemoral graft, it's outside the normal blood flow pathway.

After creating a graft tunnel between the axillary and femoral arteries, the surgeon positions the synthetic graft and anastomoses it to the axillary artery and one or both femoral arteries.

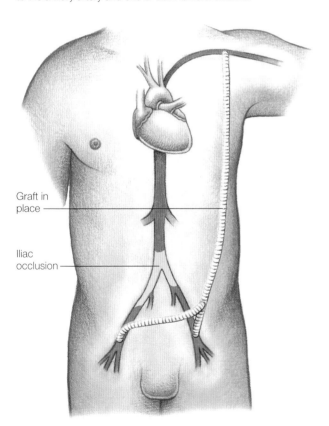

Graft in place

Iliac occlusion

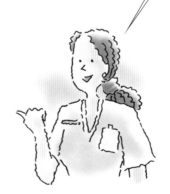

The three types of femoral bypass grafting are femoropopliteal, femorofemoral, and axillofemoral.

Thwarting graft occlusion

Graft occlusion is a potential danger after an axillofemoral bypass graft. To help prevent this problem, be careful not to position the patient on the side of the graft when providing postoperative care.

Gastric surgery

Gastric surgery is used to remove a cancerous growth or relieve an obstruction in the stomach. It's sometimes done to remove severely diseased tissue and prevent ulcer recurrence in patients with chronic ulcer disease that doesn't respond to drug therapy. The type of gastric surgery depends on the tumor's location and the extent of its spread.

Types of gastric surgery

Note: Dotted lines below show the areas removed.

Gastroduodenostomy

Also called *Billroth I,* gastroduodenostomy may be done to remove a pyloric tumor. The surgeon resects the distal one-third to one-half of the stomach and anastomoses the remaining stomach portion to the duodenum.

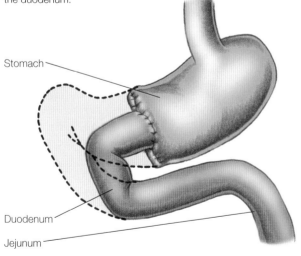

Stomach

Duodenum

Jejunum

Gastrojejunostomy

In gastrojejunostomy (Billroth II), the surgeon removes the distal portion of the antrum, anastomoses the remaining stomach to the jejunum, and closes the duodenal stump.

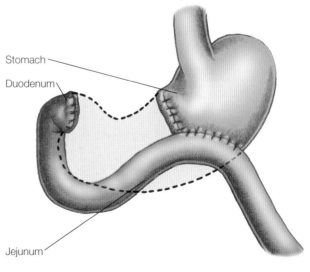

Stomach

Duodenum

Jejunum

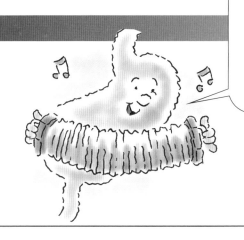

Does your stomach have you singing the blues? Types of gastric surgery include gastroduodenostomy, gastrojejunostomy, partial gastric resection, and total gastrectomy.

Partial gastric resection

For a tumor in a defined stomach area, the surgeon performs partial gastric resection by removing the diseased stomach portion and attaching the remaining stomach to the jejunum.

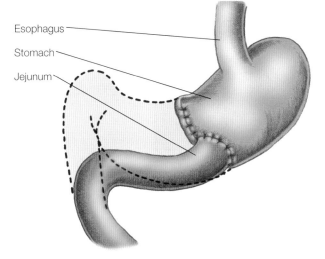

Esophagus

Stomach

Jejunum

Total gastrectomy

Total gastrectomy may be done if the tumor is in the cardia or high in the fundus. The surgeon removes the entire stomach and attaches the lower end of the esophagus to the jejunum (esophagojejunostomy) at the entrance to the small intestine.

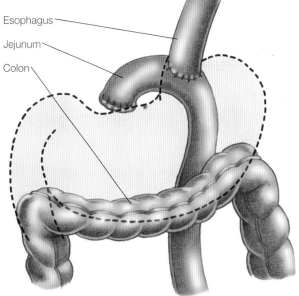

Esophagus

Jejunum

Colon

Heart transplantation

In heart transplantation, the surgeon replaces a diseased or damaged heart with a healthy donor heart. It's the treatment of choice for patients with end-stage cardiac disease (such as severe cardiomyopathy or severe ischemic or valvular heart disease) who have a poor prognosis, an estimated survival of 6 to 12 months, and a poor quality of life.

Two transplantation techniques are available — orthotopic and heterotopic. Both require cardiopulmonary bypass.

Heart transplantation involves two surgical teams. The procurement team obtains the donor heart and the recipient team transplants the donor heart into the recipient patient.

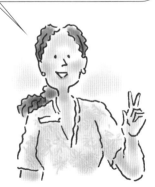

Removing the recipient's heart

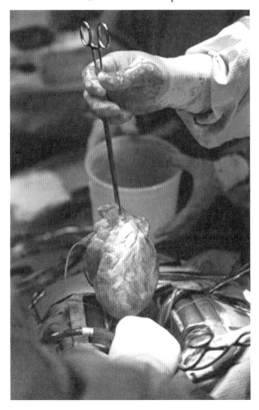

Orthotopic heart transplantation

In this most common procedure, the surgeon removes the recipient's heart and implants the donor heart at the recipient's vena cava and pulmonary veins.

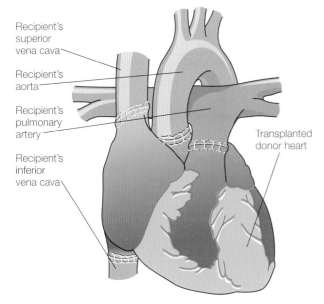

Recipient's superior vena cava

Recipient's aorta

Recipient's pulmonary artery

Recipient's inferior vena cava

Transplanted donor heart

Heterotopic heart transplantation

This rarely performed technique (also called the *piggyback method*) leaves the recipient's heart in place. The surgeon places the donor heart in the recipient's chest, in front of and to the right of the recipient's heart.

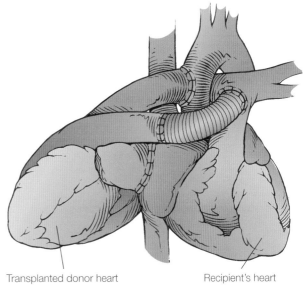

Transplanted donor heart

Recipient's heart

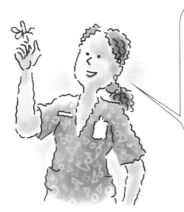

Remember — a transplanted heart has no connection to the patient's nervous system. This means atropine is useless in treating symptomatic bradycardia. Use transcutaneous pacing instead.

Hernia repair

A hernia occurs when all or part of a viscus protrudes from its normal location. Most hernias are protrusions of a part of the abdominal wall.

Hernias may be corrected by herniorrhaphy or hernioplasty, using either the open or laparoscopic approach.

Common hernia sites

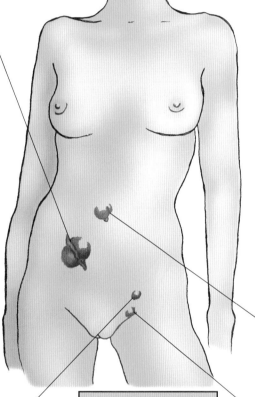

Incisional hernia

Incisional (ventral) hernia develops at a previous surgery site—usually along vertical incisions. It may be caused by abdominal wall weakness from infection or impaired wound healing. Hernia palpation may reveal several defects in the surgical scar.

To repair an incisional hernia, the surgeon pulls together abdominal wall layers without creating tension. If this isn't possible, he closes the opening with Teflon, Marlex mesh, or tantalum mesh.

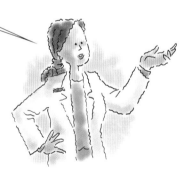

A strangulated hernia can impede normal blood flow and peristalsis, possibly causing intestinal obstruction and necrosis. A strangulated or necrotic hernia requires immediate bowel resection.

Inguinal hernia

Inguinal hernia can be direct or indirect. A *direct* inguinal hernia results from a weakness in the fascial floor of the inguinal canal. An *indirect* inguinal hernia causes abdominal viscera to protrude through the inguinal ring and follow the spermatic cord (in men) or round ligament (in women). An inguinal hernia may become incarcerated or strangulated.

Femoral hernia

Femoral hernia occurs where the femoral artery passes into the femoral canal. Typically, a fatty deposit within the femoral canal enlarges, eventually creating a hole big enough to accommodate part of the peritoneum and bladder.

A femoral hernia appears as a swelling or bulge at the pulse point of the femoral artery. Usually, it's a soft, pliable, reducible, nontender mass. It may become incarcerated or strangulated.

Most umbilical hernias in neonates close spontaneously, and surgery is done only if the hernia lasts longer than 5 years. Until the hernia closes, the affected area may be taped, bound, or supported with a truss to relieve symptoms.

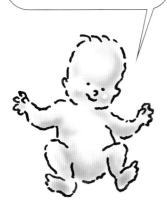

Umbilical hernia

An umbilical hernia results from abnormal muscular structures around the umbilical cord. It's common in neonates and in women who are obese or who have had several pregnancies. In severe congenital umbilical hernia, abdominal viscera protrude outside the body. This condition requires immediate repair.

Herniorrhaphy

Herniorrhaphy is used to return the protruding intestine to the abdominal cavity and repair the abdominal wall defect. To repair an indirect inguinal hernia, the surgeon makes a transverse suprainguinal incision and dissects surrounding structures to expose the hernia sac. He dissects the sac away from the spermatic cord until the neck of the hernia is visible. Then he opens the sac and returns its abdominal contents to the peritoneal cavity. He places a purse-string suture in the neck of the sac and excises the remaining hernia portion.

Hernioplasty

Used for more extensive hernias, hernioplasty reinforces the weakened area around the repair with plastic, steel, or tantalum mesh or wire. The mesh plug technique is preferred for repairing initial and recurrent inguinal hernias.

Indirect inguinal hernia repair

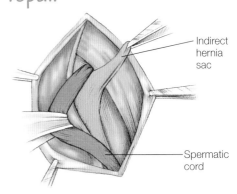

Indirect hernia sac

Spermatic cord

Mesh plug for hernia repair

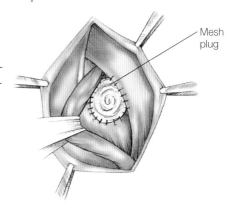

Mesh plug

Hip joint fracture repair

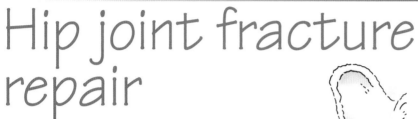

Most hip joint fractures occur in the neck of the femur (called *intracapsular fractures*) or the intertrochanteric region of the femur (called *extracapsular fractures*). Most common in elderly patients, femoral neck and intertrochanteric fractures usually require open reduction and internal fixation.

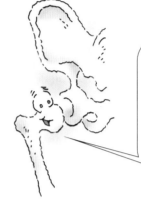

> Hip joint fractures are most common in the neck or intertrochanteric regions of the femur.

Repairing a femoral neck fracture

Before surgery, a femoral neck fracture is reduced by closed reduction. The reduction is maintained through patient positioning and traction adjustment on the operating room table.

During surgery, the surgeon makes a lateral incision over the greater trochanter and dissects subcutaneous and fascial tissue to expose the femoral neck. Then he inserts guide pins into the femoral head and inserts screws of the appropriate length over the pins. Once the screws are placed, he compresses the anterior screws and then the posterior screws.

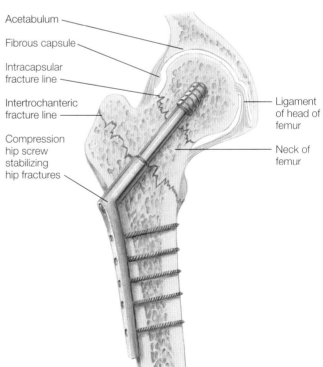

Acetabulum

Fibrous capsule

Intracapsular fracture line

Intertrochanteric fracture line

Compression hip screw stabilizing hip fractures

Ligament of head of femur

Neck of femur

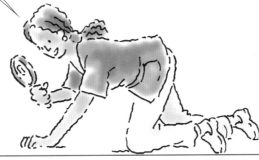

Internal fixation devices for hip fracture

The choice of internal fixation devices (screws and plates) for hip fracture repair depends on the type of fracture. The cannulated screw fixation device is used for nondisplaced femoral neck fractures.

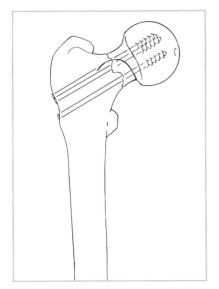

Cannulated screw fixation

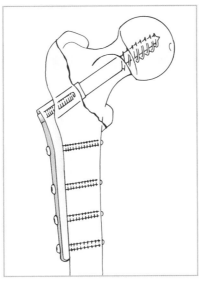

Compression hip screw and side plate

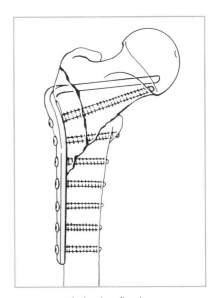

Blade plate fixation

Op sight

Hysterectomy

Hysterectomy (uterus removal) may be performed using the abdominal, vaginal, or laparoscopic-assisted approach. Hysterectomies fall into four classifications.

Total abdominal hysterectomy

Note: The dark lines below show the incision lines for uterus and cervix removal.

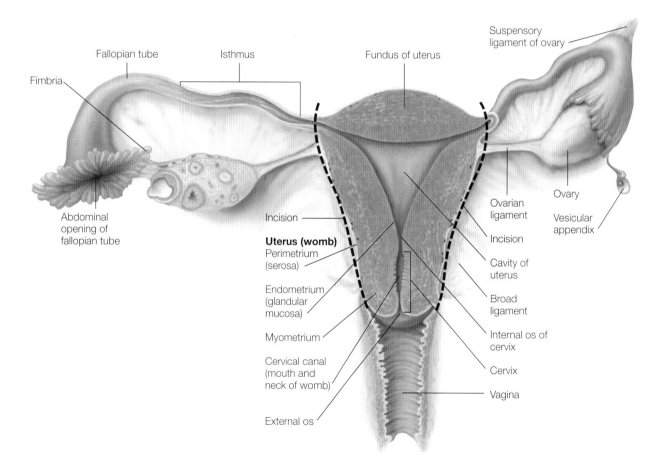

Fallopian tube

Isthmus

Fundus of uterus

Suspensory ligament of ovary

Fimbria

Abdominal opening of fallopian tube

Incision

Uterus (womb)
Perimetrium (serosa)

Endometrium (glandular mucosa)

Myometrium

Cervical canal (mouth and neck of womb)

External os

Ovarian ligament

Incision

Cavity of uterus

Broad ligament

Internal os of cervix

Cervix

Vagina

Ovary

Vesicular appendix

Hysterectomy classifications

1 **Subtotal hysterectomy:** The surgeon removes the entire uterus except the cervix (rarely done today).

2 **Total abdominal hysterectomy:** The surgeon removes the entire uterus and cervix. He makes a transverse or midline incision and dissects through the abdominal layers until the uterus is exposed. Then he removes the uterus and accompanying structures (as necessary) and closes the wound.

3 **Panhysterectomy:** The surgeon removes the entire uterus, along with the ovaries and fallopian tubes (salpingo-oophorectomy).

4 **Radical hysterectomy:** The surgeon removes the entire uterus; ovaries; fallopian tubes; adjoining ligaments and lymph nodes; and upper third of the vagina and surrounding tissues. This procedure requires an abdominal approach.

Vaginal approach

In the vaginal approach, the surgeon makes an incision inside the vagina, above but near the cervix. He excises the uterus and removes it through the vaginal canal.

In a laparoscopic-assisted vaginal hysterectomy, the surgeon makes a small incision in the umbilicus for insertion of the laparoscope (with attached camera). He insufflates the abdomen with carbon dioxide, which allows him to view the structures. Then he inserts the laparoscope and may make additional incisions to pass the instruments and excise the uterus. After excising the uterus and accompanying structures, he removes them vaginally and closes the incision.

Vaginal hysterectomy

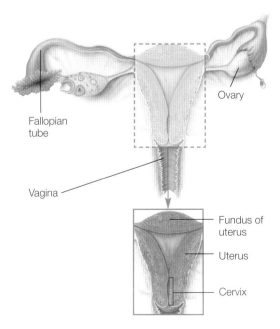

Ovary

Fallopian tube

Vagina

Fundus of uterus

Uterus

Cervix

Viewing a laparoscopic-assisted vaginal hysterectomy

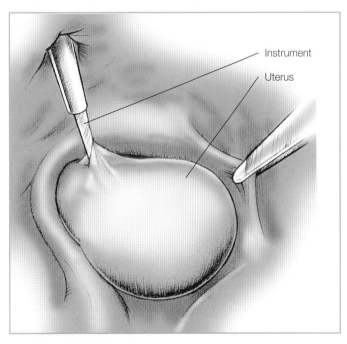

Instrument

Uterus

Op sight

Joint replacement

Total or partial replacement of a joint (arthroplasty) with a synthetic prosthesis is used to restore joint mobility and stability, relieve pain, and increase the patient's independence. Advances in surgical techniques and prosthetic devices have made joint replacement a common treatment for severe arthritis; other degenerative joint disorders that cause fragmentation, thinning, and erosion of joint cartilage; and extensive joint trauma.

Total knee replacement

> Major extremity joints can be replaced with prostheses. Knees and hips are the most commonly replaced joints.

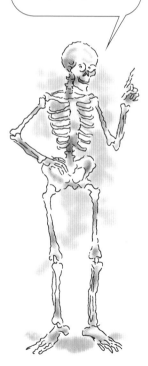

With the patient in a supine position with his knee flexed slightly, a tourniquet is applied to the upper thigh. The surgeon makes a midline incision about 4″ (10.2 cm) above the patella, enters the joint capsule medially, and exposes the tibiofemoral joint. He resects and sizes the tibia and femur and then reams the tibia. Then he reassesses tibial size, sizes the patella, and inserts the knee prosthesis (with or without bone cement).

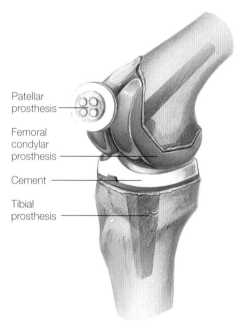

Patellar prosthesis

Femoral condylar prosthesis

Cement

Tibial prosthesis

Total hip replacement

With the patient in the lateral position, the surgeon makes an incision to expose the hip joint. He incises or excises the hip capsule and reams and shapes the acetabulum to accept the socket of the prosthesis. He repeats the process on the head of the femur for the ball of the prosthesis.

Next, he cements the femoral head prosthesis in place to articulate with a cup, which he cements into the deepened acetabulum. To avoid using cement, he may implant a prosthesis with a porous coating that promotes bony ingrowth.

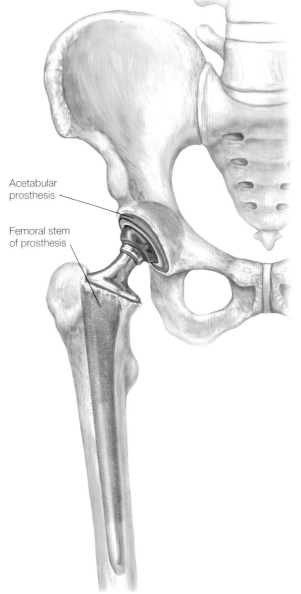

Acetabular prosthesis

Femoral stem of prosthesis

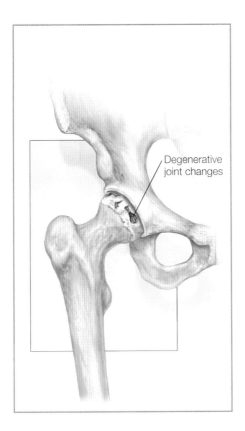

Degenerative joint changes

Kidney transplantation

In kidney transplantation, a healthy kidney is removed from a donor and implanted in a patient with nonfunctional kidneys. As with other transplantations, two surgical teams are involved — one team procures the donor kidney and the other team implants it into the recipient. Sometimes, simultaneous pancreas-kidney (SPK) transplantation is performed, in which a pancreas is transplanted along with a kidney.

Kidney transplantation site and vascular connections

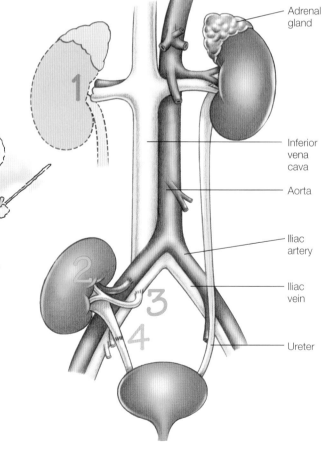

The diseased kidney is removed, and the renal artery and vein are ligated.

The donor kidney is placed in the recipient's iliac fossa.

Next, the renal artery of the donor kidney is sutured to the recipient's iliac artery and the renal vein of the donor kidney is sutured to his iliac vein.

Then the ureter of the donor kidney is sutured to the recipient's bladder or ureter.

Adrenal gland

Inferior vena cava

Aorta

Iliac artery

Iliac vein

Ureter

SPK transplantation

The donor pancreas is anastomosed using the systemic bladder technique.

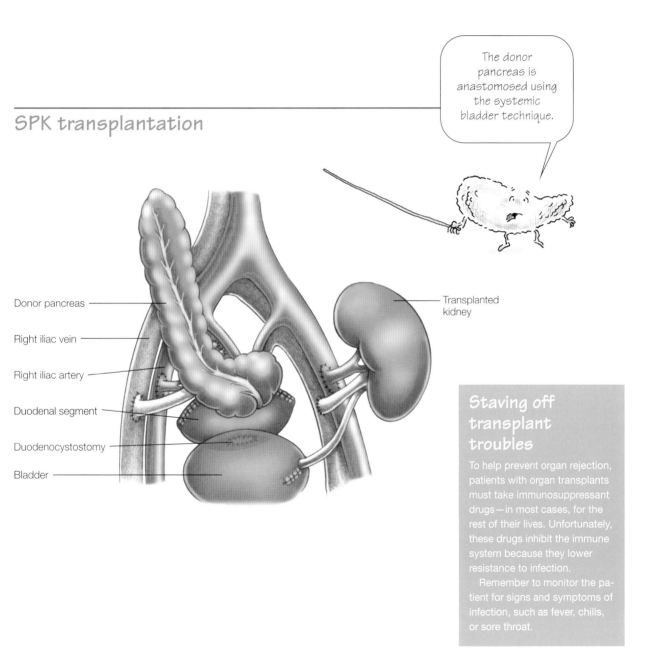

Donor pancreas

Right iliac vein

Right iliac artery

Duodenal segment

Duodenocystostomy

Bladder

Transplanted kidney

Staving off transplant troubles

To help prevent organ rejection, patients with organ transplants must take immunosuppressant drugs—in most cases, for the rest of their lives. Unfortunately, these drugs inhibit the immune system because they lower resistance to infection.

Remember to monitor the patient for signs and symptoms of infection, such as fever, chills, or sore throat.

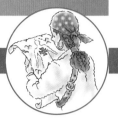

Op sight

Laminectomy

In laminectomy, the surgeon removes one or more of the bony laminae that cover the vertebrae. The procedure can be done using either a conventional or a minimally invasive technique (such as micro-diskectomy).

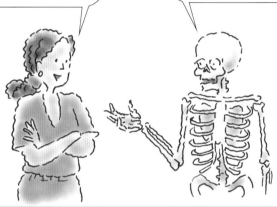

Laminectomy is most commonly performed to relieve pressure on the spinal cord or spinal nerve roots caused by a herniated intervertebral disk.

It's also done to treat a compression fracture, vertebral dislocation, or spinal cord tumor.

Tracing pain from a herniated disk

Note: The arrows in this illustration show the perceived pain path along the spinal nerve in a patient with a herniated intervertebral disk.

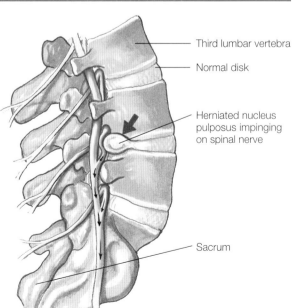

Third lumbar vertebra

Normal disk

Herniated nucleus pulposus impinging on spinal nerve

Sacrum

Removing disk material during lumbar laminectomy

In a lumbar laminectomy, the surgeon makes a midline vertical incision and strips the fascia and muscles off the bony laminae. Then he removes one or more sections of laminae to expose the spinal defect. If the disk is herniated, he removes part or all of it.

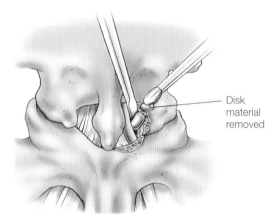

Disk material removed

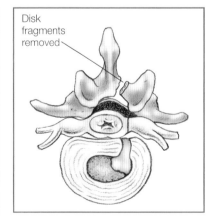

The surgical microscope magnifies the nerve root and surrounding structures.

Microdiskectomy

Microdiskectomy is a minimally invasive procedure performed with the aid of a surgical microscope. In a lumbar microdiskectomy, the surgeon makes a small incision in the patient's back for passage of the microscope and microsurgical instruments. Using a microsurgical grasping device, he carefully retracts the nerve root and removes disk fragments.

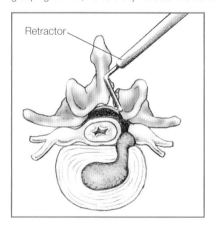

Retractor

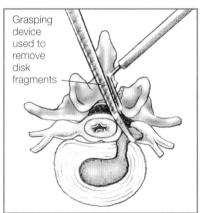

Grasping device used to remove disk fragments

Disk fragments removed

Op sight

Liver transplantation

Patients with life-threatening end-stage hepatic disease who don't respond to other treatments may undergo liver transplantation.

After the procurement team delivers the donor liver, the recipient team surgeon makes a midline abdominal incision and bilateral subcostal incisions in the recipient. He dissects underlying tissue until the liver is exposed and then removes the diseased liver.

The donor liver is flushed with cold lactated Ringer's solution and placed in the recipient's right upper abdomen. To revascularize it, the surgeon performs end-to-end anastomoses of the vena cava, portal vein, and hepatic artery. Then he performs biliary reconstruction with end-to-end anastomosis of the donor and recipient common bile ducts and inserts a T tube.

If end-to-end anastomosis can't be done, an end-to-side anastomosis is made between the common bile duct of the donor liver and a loop (Roux-en-Y portion) of the recipient's jejunum. With this procedure, a T tube isn't used and bile drainage is internal. The surgeon places the surgical drains and closes the wound.

Transplanting a liver

Roux-en-Y hepatojejunostomy

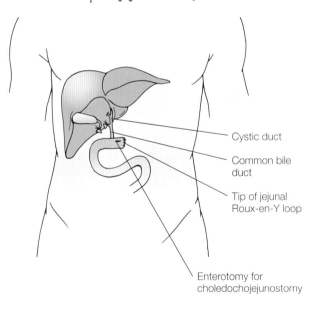

Cystic duct

Common bile duct

Tip of jejunal Roux-en-Y loop

Enterotomy for choledochojejunostomy

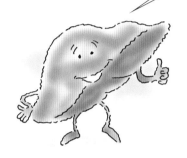

Because of the liver's ability to regenerate, liver transplantation has evolved to include both cadaver donor and living-related donor transplants.

Final appearance of transplanted liver

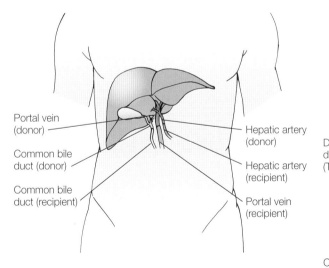

Portal vein (donor)

Common bile duct (donor)

Common bile duct (recipient)

Hepatic artery (donor)

Hepatic artery (recipient)

Portal vein (recipient)

Final closure and surgical drain placement

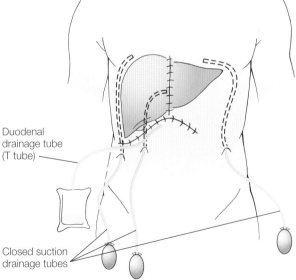

Duodenal drainage tube (T tube)

Closed suction drainage tubes

Prostatectomy

Prostatectomy is used to remove all or part of the prostate gland. Radical prostatectomy is a treatment option for patients with early-stage prostate cancer. Total or partial prostatectomy may be used in patients with significant obstructive benign prostatic hyperplasia. This procedure removes diseased or obstructive tissue and restores urine flow through the urethra.

Prostatectomy techniques include transurethral resection of the prostate (TURP), and suprapubic, retropubic, or perineal prostatectomy.

Prostatectomy techniques

TURP

With the patient in the lithotomy position, the surgeon introduces a resectoscope into the urethra and advances it to the prostate. He instills a clear, isotonic nonelectrolytic irrigating solution (such as 1.5% glycine), visualizes the obstruction, and uses the resectoscope's cutting loop to resect prostatic tissue and restore the urethral opening.

Resectoscope

Hypertrophied prostate being cut

Bladder

Suprapubic prostatectomy

With the patient in the supine position, the surgeon makes a horizontal incision above the pubic symphysis. He instills fluid into the bladder to distend it, makes a small incision in the bladder wall to expose the prostate, and shells out the obstructive prostatic tissue from the bed using his finger. Then he ligates bleeding points and usually inserts a suprapubic drainage tube and Penrose drain.

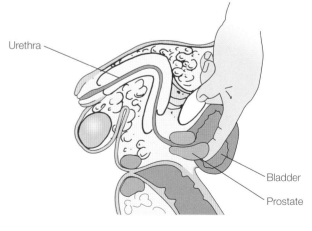

Urethra

Bladder

Prostate

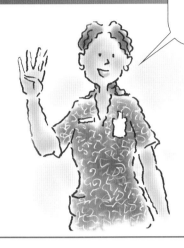

Depending on the disease, one of four prostatectomy techniques may be used.

Retropubic prostatectomy

With the patient in the supine position, the surgeon makes a horizontal suprapubic incision and approaches the prostate from between the bladder and pubic arch. After making another incision in the prostatic capsule, he removes the obstructive tissue. Usually, he inserts a suprapubic tube and Penrose drain after bleeding is controlled.

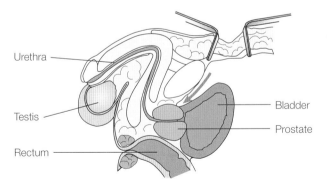

Perineal prostatectomy

With the patient in an exaggerated lithotomy position with his knees drawn up against his chest, the surgeon makes an inverted U-shaped incision in the perineum and removes the entire prostate and seminal vesicles. Then he anastomoses the urethra to the bladder and closes the incision, leaving a Penrose drain in place.

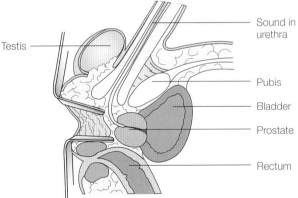

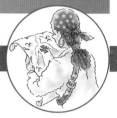

Op sight

Thoracotomy

Thoracotomy — a surgical incision into the thoracic cavity — is performed to locate and examine abnormalities (such as tumors, bleeding sites, or thoracic injuries), to take a biopsy, or to remove diseased lung tissue. Thoracotomy may involve one of three approaches — median sternotomy, anterolateral, or posterolateral.

After making the incision, the surgeon spreads the patient's ribs and exposes the lung area for excision. He may then perform pneumonectomy, lobectomy, segmental resection, or wedge resection.

Thoracoscopy may be used to confirm the diagnosis of malignant tissue or lung tumor before thoracotomy.

Types of thoracotomy

Pneumonectomy

In pneumonectomy, the surgeon excises the entire lung. After ligating and severing the pulmonary arteries, he clamps the mainstem bronchus leading to the affected lung, divides it, and closes it with nonabsorbable sutures or staples. Then he removes the lung. To ensure an airtight closure, he places a pleural flap over the bronchus.

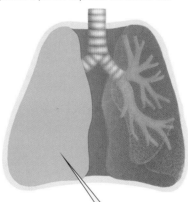

After removing the lung, the surgeon severs the phrenic nerve on the affected side and waits for air pressure in the cavity to stabilize.

Lobectomy

In lobectomy, the surgeon removes one of the five lung lobes. He resects the affected lobe and then ligates and severs the appropriate arteries, veins, and bronchial passages.

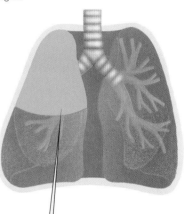

In lobectomy, the surgeon may insert one or two chest tubes for drainage and to aid lung reexpansion.

memory board

Thinking of **MAP** can help you remember the three approaches used for thoracotomy:
Median sternotomy
Anterolateral
Posterolateral.

Thoracoscopy with a video view

An invasive procedure, thoracoscopy uses a video-assisted fiber-optic endoscope to examine the thoracic cavity. Besides allowing the surgical team to visualize the visceral and parietal pleura, it may be used to perform laser procedures and wedge resection and clot evacuation or to assess pleural effusion, tumor growth, emphysema, and inflammatory and other conditions that would predispose the patient to pneumothorax. Biopsies of the pleura, mediastinal lymph nodes, and lungs can also be confirmed through thoracoscopy.

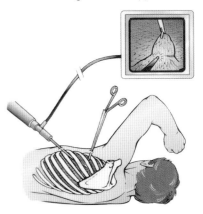

Segmental resection

In segmental resection, the surgeon removes one or more lung segments. He excises the affected segment and ligates and severs the appropriate artery, vein, and bronchus. Then he inserts a chest tube to aid lung reexpansion.

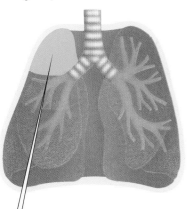

Segmental resection preserves more functional lung tissue than lobectomy.

Wedge resection

In wedge resection, the surgeon removes a small lung portion without regard to segments. He clamps and excises the affected area and then sutures it. Then he inserts a chest tube to aid lung reexpansion.

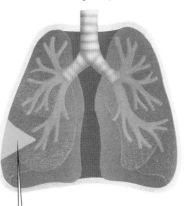

Although wedge resection preserves more functional tissue than other lung excision techniques, it can treat only a small, well-circumscribed lesion.

Protecting the pneumonectomy patient

Here are some tips to help ensure a smooth postoperative recovery for a patient who's had a pneumonectomy:
- Be aware that the chest tube is for drainage only, not reexpansion.
- Make sure the patient lies only on his back or on the operative side. Otherwise, fluid could drain into the unaffected lung if the sutured bronchus opens.
- Stay alert for bronchial stump leakage.
- Keep in mind that pneumonectomy may cause pulmonary vasculature changes that lead to atrial enlargement. As a result, atrial arrhythmias may occur.

Op sight

Thyroid surgery

Thyroidectomy—removal of all or part of the thyroid gland—is used to treat hyperthyroidism, thyroid cancer, and respiratory obstruction caused by goiter.

Incision line for thyroid surgery

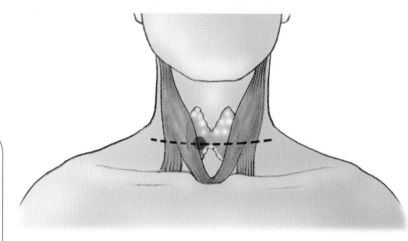

> In thyroid surgery, the surgeon fully extends the patient's neck and determines the incision line by measuring bilaterally from each clavicle.

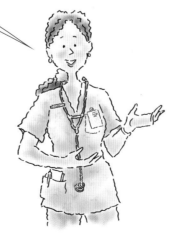

Dissecting diseased thyroid tissue

After making an incision, the surgeon cuts through skin, fascia, and muscle and raises skin flaps from the strap muscles. He separates these muscles midline, revealing the thyroid's isthmus, and then ligates the thyroid artery and veins to control bleeding. Next, he locates and visualizes the laryngeal nerves, parathyroid glands, and thyroid gland.

Then he dissects and removes the diseased thyroid tissue, avoiding nearby structures. After inserting a Penrose drain or wound drainage device, he closes the wound.

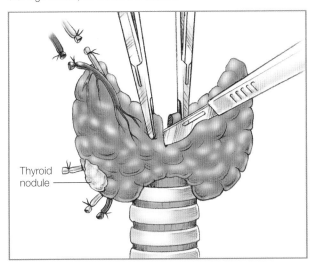

Thyroid nodule

Thyroid dissection

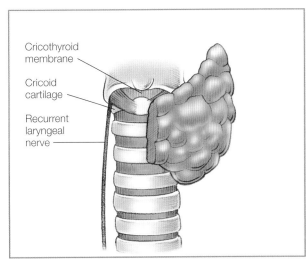

Cricothyroid membrane

Cricoid cartilage

Recurrent laryngeal nerve

Diseased lobe removal

Urinary diversion

Urinary diversion provides an alternative urine excretion route when a disease or disorder impedes normal urine flow through the bladder. The procedure may involve either a cutaneous method, such as an ileal conduit — the preferred and most common procedure for diverting urine through an ileal segment to a stoma on the abdomen — or a continent method. Continent urinary diversions include the Indiana pouch, continent ileal reservoir (Kock pouch), and modified Kock pouch. Each of these procedures begins with a cystectomy.

Creating an ileal conduit

To create an ileal conduit, the surgeon excises a segment of the ileum and closes the two resulting ends. Then he dissects the ureters from the bladder and anastomoses them to the ileal segment. He closes one end of the ileal segment with sutures and brings the opposite end through the abdominal wall to form a stoma.

Because urine empties continuously, the patient must wear a collecting device or pouch after the procedure.

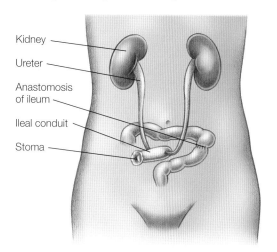

Kidney

Ureter

Anastomosis of ileum

Ileal conduit

Stoma

Continent urinary diversions

Indiana pouch

To create an Indiana pouch, the surgeon uses a segment of the small bowel or colon to form an internal pouch. He tunnels the ureters through the colon segment used to construct the pouch.

Because the pouch is internal and can hold urine without leakage, the patient won't need to use an external appliance after the surgery. However, he'll need to catheterize the abdominal opening intermittently to empty the pouch.

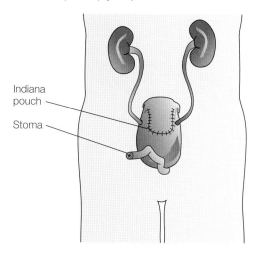

Indiana pouch

Stoma

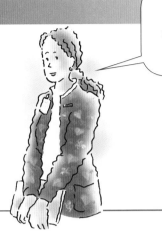

When urine flow is impeded, a urinary diversion is the answer.

Continent ileal reservoir

To create a continent ileal reservoir (Kock pouch), the surgeon forms an internal pouch from a segment of the small bowel or colon. He implants the ureters into the sides of the pouch, with each ureter intussuscepted to create a nipple valve. Then he brings the efferent ureter and nipple valve to the skin surface of the anterior abdomen as a stoma and to prevent urine leakage from the pouch. The afferent ureter and nipple valve prevent urine reflux.

Because the pouch is internal and can hold urine without leakage, the patient won't need to use an external appliance. However, he'll need to catheterize the abdominal opening intermittently to empty the pouch.

Modified Kock pouch

To create a modified Kock pouch, the surgeon modifies a continent ileal reservoir so that both ureters and the urethra connect to it. This eliminates the need for an abdominal wall opening and helps preserve the patient's body image; however, unless the lower portion of the bladder can be spared, continence depends solely on the urethra and external sphincter. For this reason, the procedure is usually done only in men because their longer urethra permits better external sphincter control.

Internal pouch drainage relies on passive emptying when the external sphincter is relaxed as well as on abdominal straining. If these techniques aren't sufficient, the patient must learn to perform intermittent self-catheterization.

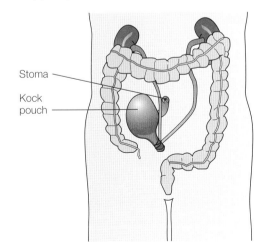

Stoma

Kock pouch

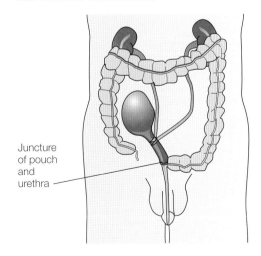

Juncture of pouch and urethra

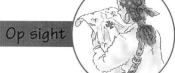

Op sight

Valvular surgery

Disease or disruption can occur in any of the four heart valves—aortic, mitral, pulmonic, or tricuspid. Surgery may be necessary if valve disease causes severe symptoms. Several procedures are available, including commissurotomy, valve repair, valve replacement, and minimally invasive valve surgery.

memory board

SIP stands for the three types of mechanical disruptions that can affect the heart valves:

Stenosis of the valve opening

Incomplete valve closure

Prolapse of the valve.

Superior view of the heart with valves

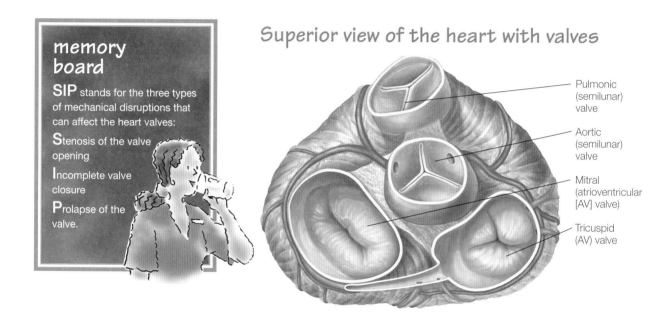

Pulmonic (semilunar) valve

Aortic (semilunar) valve

Mitral (atrioventricular [AV] valve)

Tricuspid (AV) valve

Commissurotomy

In a commissurotomy, the surgeon incises fused mitral valve leaflets and removes calcium deposits to improve valve mobility.

Valve repair

In valve repair, the surgeon resects or patches valve leaflets, stretches or shortens chordae tendineae, or places a ring in a dilated annulus (annuloplasty). Valve repair avoids the complications associated with prosthetic valves.

Valve replacement

In valve replacement, the patient's diseased valve is replaced with a mechanical or biological valve. Various types of prosthetic valves are available. Usually, valve replacement is performed through a median sternotomy.

    The surgeon splits the sternum from the manubrium to below the xiphoid process using a sternal saw. Then he spreads the ribs to expose the pericardium. The patient is placed on cardio-pulmonary bypass. After visualizing the valve, the surgeon removes the leaflets and other valve structures. He prepares the prosthetic valve and places sutures around the annulus and into the prosthetic valve. Next, he positions the new valve by sliding it down the suture and securing it in place. After suturing is complete and the valve is in place, the incision is closed.

Minimally invasive valve surgery

Minimally invasive surgery can be used to repair or replace an aortic or mitral valve, avoiding a large median sternotomy incision. Port access techniques may also be performed for mitral valve surgery using endovascular cardiopulmonary by-pass.

Replacing a heart valve

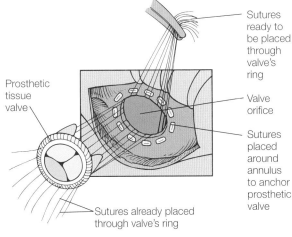

Prosthetic tissue valve

Sutures ready to be placed through valve's ring

Valve orifice

Sutures placed around annulus to anchor prosthetic valve

Sutures already placed through valve's ring

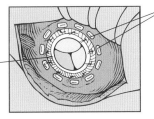

Prosthetic valve in place at end of procedure

Sutures placed around annulus to anchor prosthetic valve

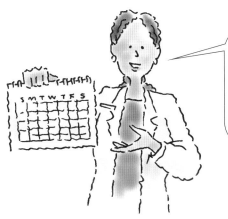

Minimally invasive valve surgery entails a shorter hospital stay, fewer postoperative complications, a smaller incision, and reduced cost.

Picturing prosthetic valves

Tilting-disk valve

The tilting-disk valve was developed as an alternative to the ball-in-cage valve. It has a hingeless design and contains open-ended, elliptical struts. These design features reduce the risk of thrombus formation. The tilting-disk valve offers an improved forward flow of blood. It also causes minimal damage to blood cells. The most common tilting-disk valve is the Medtronic Hall™ prosthesis.

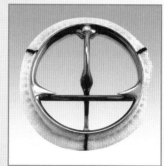

Bileaflet valve

The most commonly used prosthetic valve, a bileaflet valve consists of two semicircular leaflets that pivot on hinges. The leaflets swing partially open and are designed to close so that an acceptable amount of regurgitant blood flow is permitted. In the United States, the St. Jude Medical Valve is the most commonly inserted bileaflet valve.

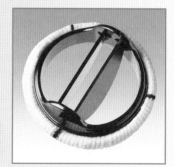

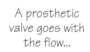

A prosthetic valve goes with the flow...

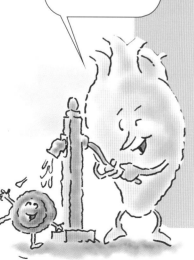

Porcine valves

A porcine valve is made using the aortic valve of a pig that's sewn to a frame called a *stent*. The stent is commonly made from a plastic composite that's covered with a polyester cloth. Porcine valves include the Carpentier-Edwards Duraflex Low-Pressure Bioprosthesis Valve and the Medtronic Hancock® II Valve.

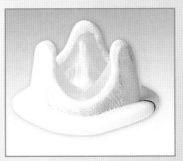 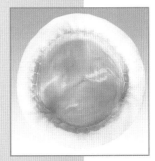

Bovine valves

A bovine valve is made from the pericardial tissue of a cow. Ionescu-Shiley constructed the first bovine valve; however, that valve has been discontinued. The Carpentier-Edwards PERIMOUNT Pericardial Bioprosthesis Valve is now widely used.

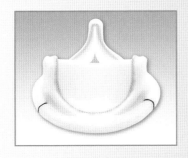

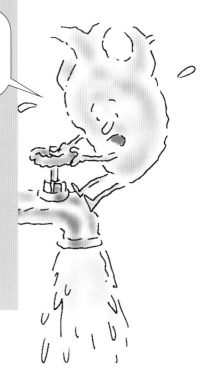

VISION QUEST

Able to label?

Label the anatomic parts and surgically created features indicated in this ileal conduit.

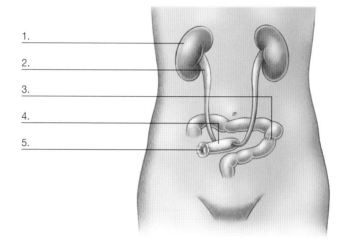

1. _____
2. _____
3. _____
4. _____
5. _____

Color my world

In this illustration of total knee replacement surgery, color the natural knee and leg structures brown and the prosthetic parts grey.

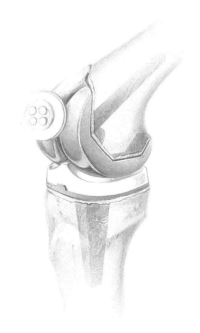

Stoma; Color my world see page 102.

Answers: Able to label? 1. Kidney, 2. Ureter, 3. Anastomosis of ileum, 4. Ileal conduit, 5.

5 Perianesthesia care

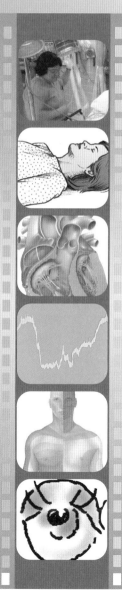

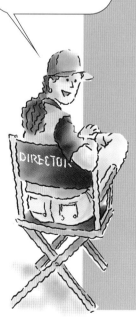

Now that your patient's surgery is completed, your role is just heating up.

- Perianesthesia nursing care basics 124
- Immediate postoperative assessment 125
- Postanesthesia complications 135
- PACU discharge criteria 145
- Vision quest 146

Perianesthesia nursing care basics

The immediate perianesthesia period starts when the patient arrives in the postanesthesia care unit (PACU), accompanied by the anesthesiologist or nurse anesthetist. During this critical phase, the patient's vital physiologic functions must be supported until the anesthetic effects wear off.

When the patient arrives in the PACU, his identity is confirmed, arrival time is documented, and the PACU nurse receives a report from the anesthesia provider.

Anesthesia provider's report

- Patient's name
- Surgical procedure performed
- Type of anesthesia used
- Vital signs trend during surgery
- Anesthetic course, including any problems and interventions
- Time when patient received reversal agents, pain medications, and other medications in the operating room
- Immediate PACU interventions needed, such as establishing correct ventilator settings or administering drugs or blood transfusions
- Estimated blood or fluid loss during surgery
- Blood and fluid replacement given during surgery
- Medical and social history (such as myocardial infarction, diabetes mellitus, stroke, asthma, hearing loss, or language barrier)
- Allergies (such as to drugs, foods, environmental factors, or latex)

Patient arrival in the PACU

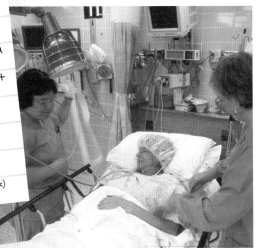

Immediate postoperative assessment

In the PACU, conduct a rapid assessment immediately after the patient arrives. Continue to perform ongoing assessments and interventions based on your findings. Remember to document your assessment findings on the PACU flow sheet, according to your facility's policy.

Body system assessment

Neurologic system

- Level of consciousness
- Orientation and ability to follow commands
- Cranial nerve function, motor function, sensation, and reflexes
- Intracranial pressure (ICP) monitoring parameters

Respiratory system

- Airway patency
- Respiratory rate and depth
- Breath sounds (note adventitious sounds)
- Chest symmetry, lung expansion, or use of accessory muscles
- Tracheal deviation from midline
- Oxygen saturation and oxygen delivery system

Cardiovascular system

- Vital signs
- Heart sounds (note presence of S_3, S_4, or murmurs)
- Hemodynamic parameters
- Cardiac rhythm
- Peripheral pulses

GI system

- Abdominal findings (such as soft, nontender, distended, or tender)
- Bowel sounds
- Nausea and vomiting
- Type and amount of drainage from drainage tubes

Musculoskeletal system

- Symmetrical body parts, proper body alignment
- Equal bilateral muscle strength, active range of motion (ROM) (note deficits or pain)

Renal system

- Fluid intake and output
- Fluid and electrolyte balance
- Type and amount of drainage from drainage tubes and catheters
- Thrill and bruit with arteriovenous (AV) fistula

Integumentary system

- Skin texture and turgor
- Skin temperature, moisture, and color
- Risk for impaired skin integrity

PACU flow sheet

The PACU flow sheet usually includes several assessment parameter tools, such as tools for assessing the patient's postanesthesia recovery, peripheral pulses, muscle strength, neurologic status, and pain.

Assess the patient using this scale until he meets discharge criteria. The maximum total score is 10. To meet discharge criteria, he must score at least an 8.

Postanesthesia recovery scoring system

Criterion	Explanation	Score
Activity	Moves four extremities voluntarily or on command	2
	Moves two extremities voluntarily or on command	1
	No movement (moves no extremities)	0
Respiration	Able to cough and deep breathe freely	2
	Dyspnea or hypoventilation	1
	Apnea	0
Circulation	Blood pressure 20% of preanesthesia level	2
	Blood pressure 21% to 49% of preanesthesia level	1
	Blood pressure 50% of preanesthesia level	0
Consciousness	Fully awake	2
	Responds to verbal stimuli (including name)	1
	No response	0
Oxygen saturation	Maintains oxygen saturation (Spo_2) > 92% on room air	2
	Needs supplemental oxygen to maintain Spo_2 > 92%	1
	Spo_2 < 92% with supplemental oxygen	0
	TOTAL SCORE:	

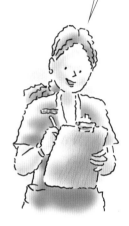

Documenting pulses

When documenting the patient's pulses, use a four-point scale from 0 to 4+.

Grading muscle strength

5/5   **Normal:** Patient moves joint through full ROM and against gravity with full resistance.

4/5   **Good:** Patient completes ROM against gravity with moderate resistance.

3/5   **Fair:** Patient completes ROM against gravity only.

2/5   **Poor:** Patient completes ROM with gravity eliminated (passive motion).

1/5   **Trace:** Patient's attempt at muscle contraction is palpable but without joint movement.

0/5   **None:** No evidence of muscle contraction is present.

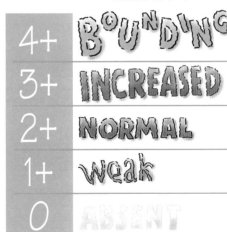

4+ BOUNDING
3+ INCREASED
2+ NORMAL
1+ weak
0 ABSENT

Assessing neurologic function

The Glasgow Coma Scale is one of several neurologic assessment tools you may use to assess the patient's neurologic function in the PACU.

Glasgow Coma Scale

A decreased score in one or more of the categories below may signal an impending neurologic crisis. To find the patient's total score, add the scores for the best response in each category.

Test	Score	Patient's response
Eye opening		
Spontaneous	4	Opens eyes spontaneously
To speech	3	Opens eyes to verbal command
To pain	2	Opens eyes to painful stimulus
None	1	Doesn't open eyes in response to stimulus
Motor response		
Obeys	6	Reacts to verbal command
Localizes	5	Identifies localized pain
Withdraws	4	Flexes and withdraws from painful stimulus
Abnormal flexion	3	Assumes a decorticate posture
Abnormal extension	2	Assumes a decerebrate posture
None	1	No response; just lies flaccid
Verbal response		
Oriented	5	Is oriented and converses
Confused	4	Is disoriented and confused
Inappropriate words	3	Replies randomly with incorrect words
Incomprehensible	2	Moans or screams
None	1	No response
TOTAL SCORE:		

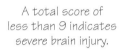

A total score of less than 9 indicates severe brain injury.

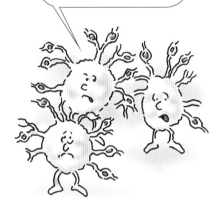

Decorticate and decerebrate postures

Decorticate

In a decorticate posture, arms are adducted and flexed, with wrists and fingers flexed on the chest. The legs are stiffly extended and internally rotated, with plantar flexion of the feet. This posture results from damage to one or both corticospinal tracts.

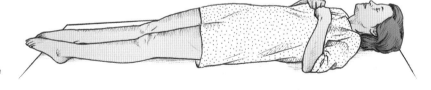

Decerebrate

In a decerebrate posture, the arms are adducted and extended, with wrists pronated and fingers flexed. The legs are stiffly extended, with plantar flexion of the feet. This posture results from damage to the upper brain stem.

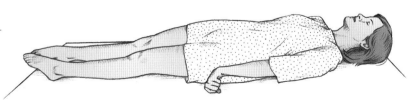

Pain rating scales

Because pain is a subjective experience, the most valid pain assessment comes from the patient. Pain assessment tools include the numeric, visual analog, and Wong-Baker FACES pain rating scales.

Your documentation should include pain assessment findings, interventions taken to manage pain (such as epidural analgesia or I.V. opioids), pain reassessment times, and effectiveness of pain management interventions.

Tools for evaluating pain in infants and children include the COMFORT scale, CRIES scale for neonatal postoperative pain assessment, and FLACC scale, which is used with children ages 2 months to 7 years.

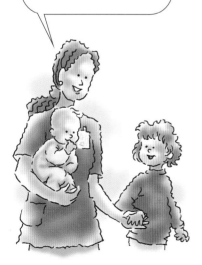

Numeric pain rating scale

The patient chooses a number from 0 (meaning no pain) to 10 (meaning the worst pain imaginable) to describe his pain level. He can either circle the number on the scale or state the number that best describes his pain.

| No pain | 0 | 1 | 2 | 3 | 4 | 5 | 6 | 7 | 8 | 9 | 10 | Pain as bad as it can be |

Visual analog pain rating scale

When using the visual analog scale, ask the patient to place a mark on the scale to indicate his pain level.

No pain |————————————————X————| Pain as bad as it can be

Wong-Baker FACES pain rating scale

A child or an adult with language difficulties may be unable to describe the pain he's feeling. If so, use this pain intensity scale. Ask him to choose the face that best represents the severity of his pain when using a scale from 0 to 10.

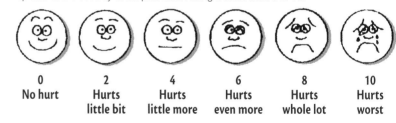

| 0 No hurt | 2 Hurts little bit | 4 Hurts little more | 6 Hurts even more | 8 Hurts whole lot | 10 Hurts worst |

memory board

Remember the mnemonic device **CRIES** when assessing pain in neonates (age 0 to 6 months):
Crying (high-pitched)
Requires oxygen for oxygen saturation <95%
Increased vital signs (blood pressure and heart rate)
Expression (grimace)
Sleepless.

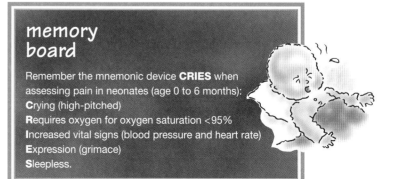

> Catch the wave! Here are the components of a normal arterial waveform.

Hemodynamic monitoring

Hemodynamic monitoring provides crucial information about the patient's cardiac function and allows the health care team to determine if interventions have been effective. Hemodynamic measurements include:
- blood pressure
- cardiac output
- intracardiac pressures
- mixed venous oxygen saturation.

Arterial pressure monitoring

Normal arterial blood pressure produces a characteristic waveform representing ventricular systole and diastole.

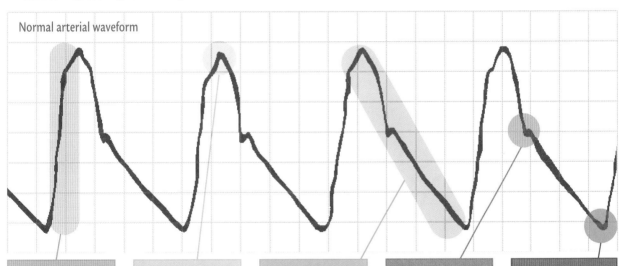

Normal arterial waveform

Anacrotic limb	Systolic peak	Dicrotic limb	Dicrotic notch	End diastole
The *anacrotic limb* marks the waveform's initial upstroke, which occurs as blood is rapidly ejected from the ventricle through the open aortic valve into the aorta.	Arterial pressure then rises sharply, resulting in the *systolic peak*—the waveform's highest point.	As blood continues into the peripheral vessels, arterial pressure falls and the waveform begins a downward trend, called the *dicrotic limb*. Arterial pressure usually keeps falling until pressure in the ventricle is less than pressure in the aortic root.	When ventricular pressure is lower than aortic root pressure, the aortic valve closes. This event appears as a small notch on the waveform's downside, called the *dicrotic notch*.	When the aortic valve closes, diastole begins, progressing until aortic root pressure gradually falls to its lowest point. On the waveform, this is known as *end diastole*.

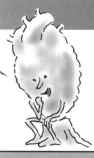

Before caring for a patient who requires PA catheterization, familiarize yourself with a basic catheter.

Come equipped

Picturing a pulmonary artery catheter

Pulmonary artery (PA) catheterization provides information about your patient's cardiovascular and pulmonary status. With a basic PA catheter, you can measure intracardiac pressure, pulmonary artery wedge pressure (PAWP), and cardiac output. More specialized PA catheters may have fiber-optic filaments for continuous mixed venous oxygen saturation measurement as well as pacing capabilities.

When your patient requires a PA catheter, your responsibilities may include assisting with insertion, caring for the insertion site and catheter, and performing hemodynamic monitoring.

Balloon inflation valve

The balloon inflation valve serves as the access point for inflating the balloon at the distal tip of the catheter for PAWP measurement.

Proximal lumen

The proximal lumen, usually blue, typically opens into the right atrium. Besides measuring right atrial pressure (RAP), it delivers the bolus injection used to measure cardiac output. It also serves as a fluid infusion route.

Distal lumen

The distal lumen, usually yellow, opens into the pulmonary artery. When attached to a transducer, it allows measurement of PA pressures and PAWP.

Thermistor

The thermistor measures core body temperature. When connected to a cardiac output monitor, it measures temperature changes related to cardiac output.

Venous infusion lumen

The venous infusion lumen is an additional lumen, which may be used for fluid administration.

Inflated balloon

The inflated balloon wedges into a branch of the pulmonary artery during PAWP measurement.

Normal PA waveforms

After insertion into a large vein (usually the subclavian, jugular, or femoral vein), a PA catheter is advanced through the vena cava into the right atrium, through the right ventricle and into a branch of the pulmonary artery. As the catheter advances through the heart chambers, the monitor shows various waveforms.

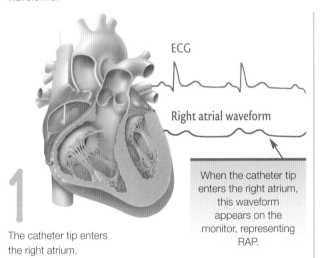

ECG

Right atrial waveform

When the catheter tip enters the right atrium, this waveform appears on the monitor, representing RAP.

1 The catheter tip enters the right atrium.

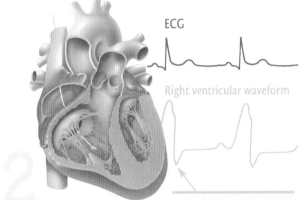

ECG

Right ventricular waveform

As the catheter tip reaches the right ventricle, you'll see a waveform with sharp systolic upstrokes and lower diastolic dips.

2 Next, the catheter tip reaches the right ventricle.

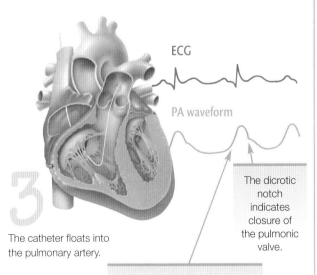

ECG

PA waveform

The dicrotic notch indicates closure of the pulmonic valve.

3 The catheter floats into the pulmonary artery.

As the catheter reaches the pulmonary artery, the upstroke of the waveform becomes smoother than that of the right ventricular waveform.

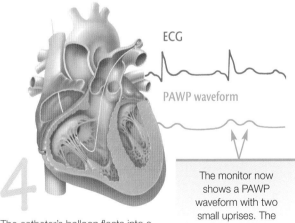

ECG

PAWP waveform

The monitor now shows a PAWP waveform with two small uprises. The balloon is then deflated and the catheter is left in the pulmonary artery.

4 The catheter's balloon floats into a distal branch of the pulmonary artery. It wedges where the vessel becomes too narrow for it to pass.

Hemodynamic parameters

Hemodynamic monitoring provides information on arterial pressure, intracardiac pressures, cardiac output, cardiac index, stroke volume, and systemic vascular resistance. To understand intracardiac pressures, picture the heart and vascular system as a continuous loop with constantly changing pressure gradients that keep blood moving.

Hemodynamic monitoring records the gradients within the vessels and heart chambers. Hemodynamic parameters provide information about cardiac function and the effectiveness of therapeutic interventions.

Parameter	Normal value
Mean arterial pressure (MAP)	▪ 70 to 105 mm Hg

$$MAP = \frac{Systolic + 2\ (Diastolic)}{3}$$

Parameter	Normal value
Central venous pressure (CVP); RAP	▪ 2 to 6 cm H_2O; 2 to 8 mm Hg
Right ventricular pressure	▪ 20 to 30 mm Hg (systolic) ▪ 0 to 8 mm Hg (diastolic)
Pulmonary artery pressure (PAP)	▪ 20 to 30 mm Hg (PA systolic) ▪ 8 to 15 mm Hg (PA diastolic) ▪ 10 to 20 mm Hg (PA mean)
PAWP	▪ 4 to 12 mm Hg
Cardiac output (CO)	▪ 4 to 8 L/minute

$$CO = Heart\ rate\ (HR) \times Stroke\ volume\ (SV)$$

Parameter	Normal value
Cardiac index (CI)	▪ 2.5 to 4 L/minute/m^2

$$CI = \frac{CO}{Body\ surface\ area\ (BSA)}$$

Parameter	Normal value
SV	▪ 60 to 100 ml/beat

$$SV = \frac{CO \times 1,000}{HR}$$

Parameter	Normal value
Stroke volume index (SVI)	▪ 33 to 47 ml/beat/m^2

$$SVI = \frac{CI \times 1,000}{HR}$$

Parameter	Normal value
Systemic vascular resistance (SVR)	▪ 800 to 1,200 dynes/sec/cm^{-5}

$$SVR = \frac{MAP - RAP}{CO} \times 80$$

Parameter	Normal value
Systemic vascular resistance index (SVRI)	▪ 1,900 to 2,400 dynes/sec/cm^{-5}/m^2

$$SVRI = \frac{MAP - RAP}{CI} \times 80$$

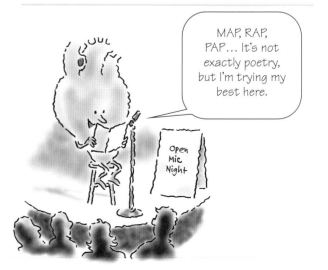

MAP, RAP, PAP... It's not exactly poetry, but I'm trying my best here.

ICP monitoring

ICP monitoring measures the pressure exerted by the brain, blood, and cerebrospinal fluid against the inside of the skull. By allowing prompt detection and intervention of problems, ICP monitoring helps avert damage caused by cerebral hypoxia and brain mass shifts.

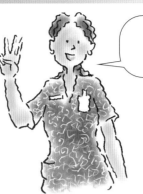

Three waveforms — A, B, and C — are used to monitor ICP.

ICP waveforms

Normal waveform

A normal ICP waveform typically has a steep upward systolic slope followed by a downward diastolic slope with a dicrotic notch. In most cases, this waveform occurs continuously and indicates an ICP between 0 and 15 mm Hg—normal pressure.

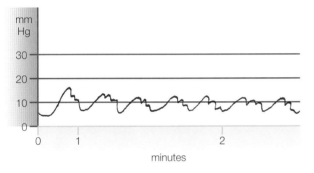

B waves

B waves, which appear sharp and rhythmic with a sawtooth pattern, occur every 1½ to 2 minutes and may reach elevations of 50 mm Hg. Their clinical significance isn't clear, but the waves correlate with respiratory changes and may occur more often with decreasing compensation.

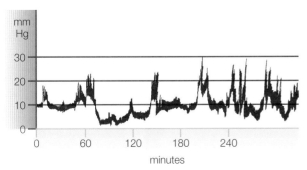

A waves

The most clinically significant ICP waveforms are A waves, which may reach elevations of 50 to 100 mm Hg, persist for 5 to 20 minutes, then drop sharply—signaling exhaustion of the brain's compliance mechanisms. Certain activities, such as sustained coughing or straining during defecation, can cause temporary intracranial pressure elevations.

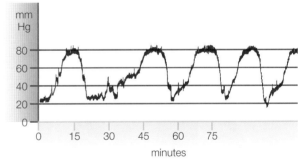

C waves

Like B waves, C waves are rapid and rhythmic, but they aren't as sharp. Clinically insignificant, they may fluctuate with respirations or systemic blood pressure changes.

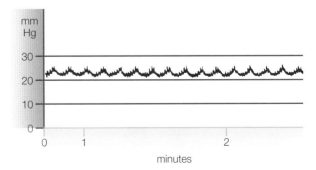

Assessing level of blockade from spinal anesthesia

Spinal anesthesia produces a sympathetic, sensory, and motor block. If your patient received spinal anesthesia, be sure to assess the downward progression of the level of blockade. Using a dermatome chart aids this assessment. Each dermatome represents a specific body area supplied with nerve fibers from an individual spinal root (cervical, thoracic, lumbar, or sacral).

Division by dermatomes

To document the patient's sensory and motor function, mentally divide his body into dermatomes, as shown here. Anatomic reference points include the nipple line at T4, xiphoid at T6, umbilicus at T10, and groin at L1.

> Use the body map below when testing sensation to determine the level of blockade from spinal anesthesia.

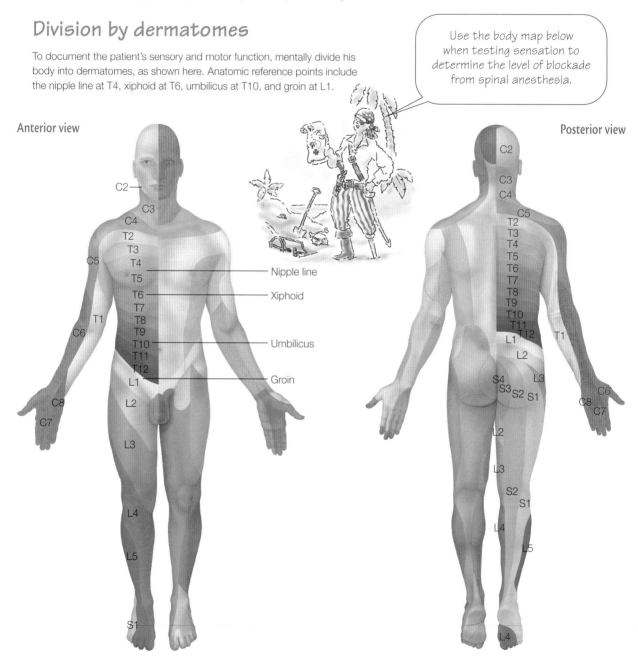

Anterior view

Posterior view

Nipple line
Xiphoid
Umbilicus
Groin

Postanesthesia complications

Postanesthesia complications include:
- respiratory complications
- cardiovascular complications
- metabolic complications
- central nervous system (CNS) depression
- pain
- nausea
- vomiting.

Respiratory complications

Potential respiratory complications include hypoventilation and laryngospasm.

Hypoventilation

Hypoventilation results from the respiratory depressant effects of inhalation anesthetics and opioids as well as the patient's splinting of painful abdominal and thoracic incisions. It's a common cause of hypoxemia in the PACU.

Interventions

- Establish and maintain a patent airway.
- Provide supplemental oxygen and ventilatory support with a bag-valve mask device, endotracheal (ET) intubation, and mechanical ventilation.
- Use the "stir-up" regimen by stimulating the patient and encouraging coughing and deep breathing.
- For hypoventilation caused by opioids or muscle relaxants, reversal agents for these drugs may be given.
- Provide effective pain management measures to relieve pain and improve ventilation.

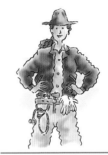

Come equipped

Bag-valve mask device

A bag-valve mask device is an inflatable handheld resuscitation bag with a reservoir that can be used with the face mask or directly attached to an ET tube or tracheostomy tube when the face mask is removed.

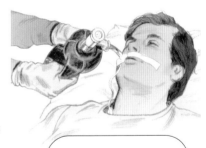

Use a bag-valve mask device to provide manually delivered ventilation of supplemental oxygen by positive pressure to patients with apnea or inadequate respirations.

Laryngospasm

Laryngospasm (spasm of the laryngeal muscle) may be *complete* (when the vocal cords close completely) or *incomplete* (when they close partially). It may result from secretions (such as blood or mucus), stimulation caused by a foreign body (such as an oral airway or a suction catheter), or vocal cord irritation from intubation or surgery. Whatever the cause, laryngospasm requires immediate intervention.

Interventions

- Immediately remove the irritation source, if possible.
- Provide gentle positive-pressure ventilation using a bag-valve mask device with 100% oxygen.
- If necessary, perform ET suctioning to remove secretions.
- If initial measures fail, the anesthesiologist may give the patient succinylcholine. Provide respiratory support with a bag-valve mask device until the drug's effects subside.
- If the patient can't maintain adequate respirations, prepare for ET intubation and mechanical ventilation.
- If ordered, give lidocaine 1.5 mg/kg I.V.
- Provide emotional support to help the patient relax.

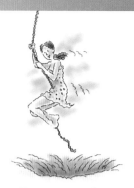

Postop pitfall
A look at laryngospasm

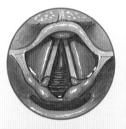

Normal larynx
Vocal cords open during normal inspiration

Laryngospasm
Sudden closure of vocal cords

Cardiovascular complications

Potential cardiovascular complications include hypotension, hypertension, and cardiac arrhythmias.

Hypotension

A common postoperative complication, hypotension may result from:
- myocardial depression and vasodilation induced by anesthetics
- decreased venous return caused by hypovolemia related to blood loss as a result of surgery
- arrhythmias
- myocardial infarction (MI)
- vasovagal response
- hypoxemia
- pain.

Interventions

- Implement interventions based on the specific cause of hypotension.
- Administer I.V. fluids and blood products to replace blood loss.
- Administer vasopressors.

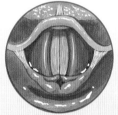

To treat postanesthesia hypotension, consider administering I.V. fluids.

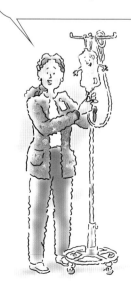

Hypertension

Postoperative hypertension usually results from preexisting hypertension, renal disease, or pain. Other causes include fluid overload, bladder distention, hypercapnia, anesthetics (such as ketamine), and naloxone (used for opioid reversal).

Interventions

- Implement interventions based on the specific cause of hypertension. For instance, give pain medication if the patient is in pain. If the patient has bladder distention, insert a urinary catheter.
- Administer antihypertensive drugs.
- Be aware that ketamine-induced hypertension may resolve without treatment.

Cardiac arrhythmias

Arrhythmias occur as a result of abnormal impulse conduction and may be classified based on the anatomic location of the electrical disturbance or according to rate. During the immediate postoperative period, arrhythmias may result from:

- myocardial depression caused by anesthetics
- hypoxemia
- pain
- hypothermia
- hypovolemia
- fluid overload
- preexisting cardiac disease or MI
- electrolyte imbalance
- fever.

Interventions

- Notify the surgeon and attending practitioner.
- Initiate cardiopulmonary resuscitation for cardiopulmonary arrest and follow basic life support and advanced cardiac life support guidelines.
- Provide supplemental oxygen and prepare for ET intubation and mechanical ventilation.
- Administer medications to treat specific arrhythmias.

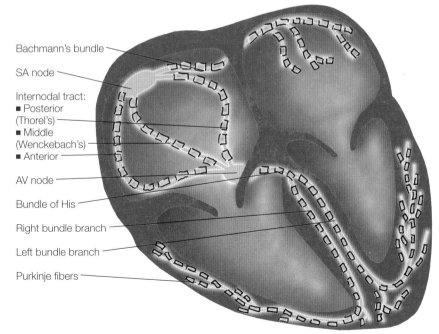

Cardiac conduction system

- Bachmann's bundle
- SA node
- Internodal tract:
  - Posterior (Thorel's)
  - Middle (Wenckebach's)
  - Anterior
- AV node
- Bundle of His
- Right bundle branch
- Left bundle branch
- Purkinje fibers

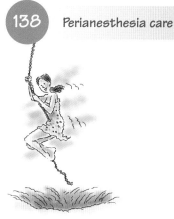

Postop pitfall

Sinus bradycardia

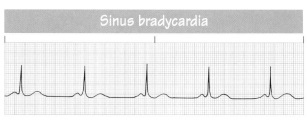

- Rhythm: regular
- Rate: < 60 beats/minute
- P wave: normal
- PR interval: 0.12 to 0.20 second

- QRS complex: 0.06 to 0.10 second
- QT interval: normal or possibly prolonged

Sinus tachycardia

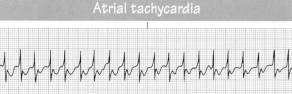

- Rhythm: regular
- Rate: 100 to 160 beats/minute
- P wave: normal
- PR interval: 0.12 to 0.20 second

- QRS complex: 0.06 to 0.10 second
- QT interval: normal or possibly shortened

Premature atrial contractions (PACs)

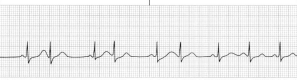

- Rhythm: irregular
- Rate: varies with underlying rhythm
- P wave: premature and abnormally shaped with PAC
- PR interval: usually within normal limits but varies with ectopic focus

- QRS complex: 0.06 to 0.10 second
- QT interval: normal (not routinely measured in PACs)

Atrial tachycardia

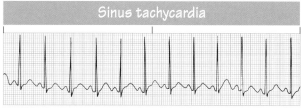

- Rhythm: regular
- Rate: 150 to 250 beats/minute; ventricular rate depends on AV conduction rates
- P wave: hidden in preceding T wave
- PR interval: not visible

- QRS complex: 0.06 to 0.10 second
- QT interval: normal or shortened

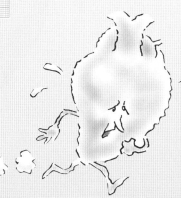

Whew! I'm getting quite a workout. In atrial tachycardia, I may beat as fast as 250 times a minute.

Atrial flutter

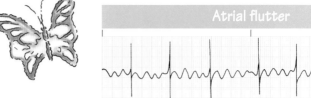

- Rhythm: atrial—regular; ventricular—typically irregular
- Rate: atrial—250 to 400 beats/minute; ventricular—usually 60 to 100 beats/minute; ventricular rate depends on degree of AV block
- P wave: classic sawtooth appearance (flutter waves)
- PR interval: not measurable
- QRS complex: 0.06 to 0.10 second
- QT interval: not measurable

Atrial fibrillation

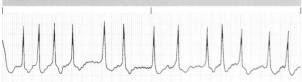

- Rhythm: irregularly irregular
- Rate: atrial—usually > 400 beats/minute; ventricular—varies
- P wave: absent; replaced by fine fibrillatory waves (f waves)
- PR interval: indiscernible
- QRS complex: 0.06 to 0.10 second
- QT interval: not measurable

Premature ventricular contractions (PVCs)

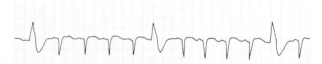

- Rhythm: irregular
- Rate: reflects the underlying rhythm
- P wave: none with PVC, but P wave present with other QRS complexes
- PR interval: unmeasurable except in underlying rhythm
- QRS complex: early, with bizarre configuration and duration of > 0.12 second; QRS complexes are normal in underlying rhythm
- QT interval: not routinely measured in PVCs

Ventricular tachycardia

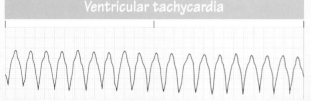

- Rhythm: regular
- Rate: atrial—can't be determined; ventricular—100 to 250 beats/minute
- P wave: absent
- PR interval: not measurable
- QRS complex: > 0.12 second; wide and bizarre
- QT interval: not measurable

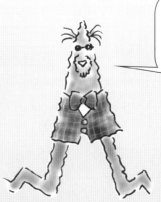

With PVCs, the QRS complex appears early with a noticeably bizarre configuration.

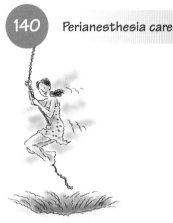

Postop pitfall

Ventricular fibrillation

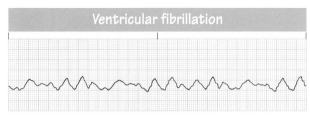

- Rhythm: chaotic
- Rate: can't be determined
- P wave: absent
- PR interval: not measurable
- QRS complex: not discernible
- QT interval: not measurable

Type I second-degree AV block

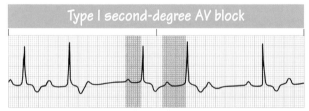

- Rhythm: atrial—regular; ventricular—irregular
- Rate: atrial—exceeds ventricular rate; both remain within normal limits
- P wave: normal
- PR interval: progressively prolonged (see shaded areas) until P wave appears without QRS complex
- QRS complex: 0.06 to 0.10 second
- QT interval: usually normal

Type II second-degree AV block

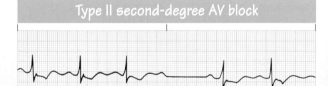

- Rhythm: atrial—regular; ventricular—irregular
- Rate: atrial—within normal limits; ventricular—slower than atrial but may be within normal limits
- P wave: normal
- PR interval: constant for conducted beats
- QRS complex: within normal limits; absent for dropped beats
- QT interval: normal

Third-degree AV block

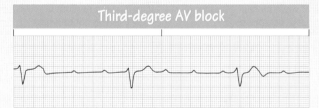

- Rhythm: regular
- Rate: atria and ventricles beat independently; atrial—60 to 100 beats/ minute; ventricular—40 to 60 beats/minute intranodal block, < 40 beats/minute infra-nodal block
- P wave: normal
- PR interval: varied; not applicable or measurable
- QRS complex: normal or widened
- QT interval: usually normal

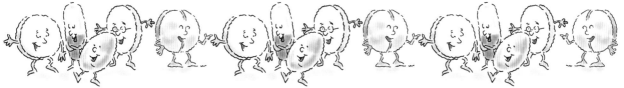

Guide to antiarrhythmic drugs

Drugs	Indications	Special considerations
Class IA antiarrhythmics		
■ disopyramide ■ procainamide ■ quinidine	■ Ventricular tachycardia (VT) ■ Atrial fibrillation ■ Atrial flutter ■ Paroxysmal atrial tachycardia (PAT)	■ Check apical pulse rate before therapy. If extreme, withhold dose and notify prescriber. ■ Use cautiously in patients with reactive airway disease such as asthma. ■ Monitor for ECG changes (widening QRS complexes, prolonged QT interval).
Class IB antiarrhythmics		
■ lidocaine ■ mexiletine ■ tocainide	■ VT ■ Ventricular fibrillation (VF)	■ IB antiarrhythmics may potentiate the effects of other antiarrhythmics. ■ Administer I.V. infusions with an infusion pump.
Class IC antiarrhythmics		
■ flecainide ■ moricizine ■ propafenone	■ VT ■ VF ■ Supraventricular arrhythmias	■ Correct electrolyte imbalances before administration. ■ Monitor ECG before and after dosage adjustments. ■ Monitor for ECG changes (widening QRS complexes, prolonged QT interval).
Class II antiarrhythmics		
■ acebutolol ■ atenolol ■ esmolol ■ propranolol	■ Atrial flutter ■ Atrial fibrillation ■ PAT	■ Monitor apical heart rate and blood pressure. ■ Abruptly stopping these drugs can exacerbate angina and trigger MI. ■ Monitor for ECG changes (prolonged PR interval). ■ Drugs may mask common signs and symptoms of shock and hypoglycemia. ■ Use with caution in patients with reactive airway disease such as asthma.

> Be careful when giving class IA antiarrhythmics to patients with asthma or other reactive airway diseases.

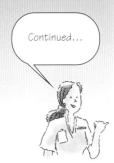

Continued…

Drugs	Indications	Special considerations
Class III antiarrhythmics		
• amiodarone • dofetilide • ibutilide • sotalol	• Life-threatening arrhythmias resistant to other antiarrhythmic drugs	• Monitor heart rate and rhythm and blood pressure for changes. • Amiodarone increases the risk of digoxin toxicity in patients also taking digoxin. • Monitor for signs and symptoms of pulmonary toxicity (nonproductive cough, dyspnea, and pleuritic chest pain), thyroid dysfunction, and vision impairment in patients taking amioda-rone. • Monitor for ECG changes (prolonged QT interval) in patients taking dofetilide, ibutilide, or sotalol.
Class IV antiarrhythmics		
• diltiazem • verapamil	• Supraventricular arrhythmias	• Monitor heart rate and rhythm and blood pressure carefully when initiating therapy or increasing dosage. • Calcium supplements may reduce effectiveness.
Miscellaneous antiarrhythmics		
• adenosine	• Paroxysmal supraventricu-lar tachycardia	• Adenosine must be given over 1 to 2 seconds, followed by 20-ml flush of normal saline solution. • Record rhythm strip during administration because adenosine may cause transient asystole or heart block.
• atropine	• Symptomatic sinus bradycardia • AV block • Asystole • Bradycardic pulseless electrical activity (PEA)	• Monitor cardiac rate and rhythm. Use drug cautiously in patients with myocardial ischemia. • Atropine isn't recommended for third-degree AV block or infranodal type II second-degree AV block. • In adults, avoid dosages below 0.5 mg because of the risk of paradoxical slowing of heart rate.
• epinephrine	• Pulseless VT • VF • Asystole • PEA	• Monitor heart rate and rhythm and blood pressure carefully because epinephrine may cause myocardial ischemia. • Don't mix I.V. dose with alkaline solutions. • Give drug into large vein to prevent irritation or extravasation at site.
• vasopressin	• VF unresponsive to defibrillation	• Monitor heart rate and rhythm. Use with caution in patients with myocardial ischemia. • Monitor for hypersensitivity reactions, especially urticaria, angioedema, and bronchoconstriction.

> Supplemental calcium may reduce the effectiveness of class IV antiarrhythmics.

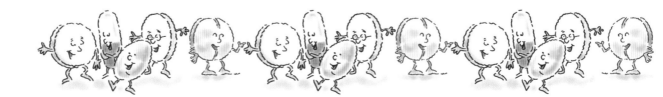

Metabolic complications

Potential metabolic complications include hypothermia and malignant hyperthermia.

Hypothermia

Postoperative hypothermia may result from the cool operating room temperature, heat loss during surgery, administration of cool irrigating or I.V. fluids, or vasodilation caused by anesthetics.

Interventions

- Provide oxygen to accommodate the increased oxygen demands caused by hypothermia.
- Remove cold, wet sheets and gown.
- Use a warming device system such as a warming blanket.
- Administer warmed fluids and blood.

Malignant hyperthermia

Malignant hyperthermia is a rare, life-threatening complication that can occur postoperatively or intraoperatively (more common). An inherited autosomal dominant disorder, it's caused by a biochemical defect in skeletal muscle and occurs when a triggering agent increases oxygen consumption and raises lactate and heat production, leading to hypermetabolism.

Signs and symptoms include:
- masseter muscle rigidity after succinylcholine administration
- hypercapnia and hypoxemia
- sudden, unexplained tachycardia and, possibly, ventricular arrhythmias
- temperature elevation (the disorder's hallmark)
- tachypnea
- respiratory and metabolic acidosis
- hyperkalemia
- myoglobinemia and myoglobinuria.

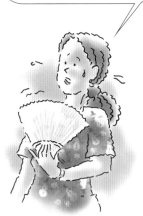

Triggers for malignant hyperthermia include volatile anesthetics and succinylcholine.

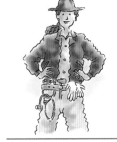

Come equipped

Warming blanket

Postoperative blankets provide even distribution of heat for safe and effective patient rewarming.

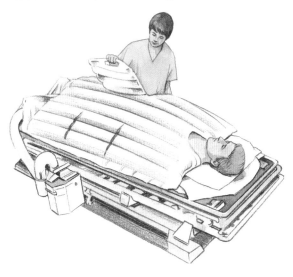

Interventions

▪ Prevention is the best treatment for malignant hyperthermia. At-risk patients should be identified preoperatively. Risk factors include:
  – personal or family history of the condition
  – history of skeletal muscle or neuromuscular disorders (such as Duchenne's muscular dystrophy)
  – history of muscle cramps or muscle rigidity with stress or exercise.

▪ If malignant hyperthermia occurs in the operating room, halt anesthesia, change anesthesia machine circuitry, and administer 100% oxygen.

▪ Call for help and obtain a malignant hyperthermia kit.

▪ Administer dantrolene, according to your facility's policy.

▪ Institute cooling measures.

▪ Correct acidosis, as indicated.

▪ Administer diuretics.

▪ Monitor the patient's vital signs, oxygen saturation, heart rate and rhythm, and serum electrolyte levels.

▪ Intervene as needed to correct arrhythmias and electrolyte imbalances.

▪ Once the patient is stabilized, prepare to transfer him to the critical care unit for additional dantrolene therapy and monitoring for potential complications (such as renal failure and disseminated intravascular coagulation).

▪ After the crisis, refer the patient and his family to the Malignant Hyperthermia Association of the United States for counseling and information on diagnostic testing.

Malignant hyperthermia kit

A malignant hyperthermia kit contains:
- dantrolene sodium 20 mg (36 vials)
- sterile water for drug dilution
- dextrose 50%
- furosemide
- calcium gluconate
- sodium bicarbonate
- regular insulin
- mannitol
- methylprednisolone
- procainamide
- I.V. cannulas (assorted sizes)
- I.V. administration sets
- three-way stopcocks
- central venous pressure sets
- blood collection tubes
- oxygen tubing and delivery devices
- arterial blood gas kit
- nasogastric tubes
- indwelling urinary catheter tray
- normal saline irrigation solution and I.V. fluids (normal saline solution) — which are removed from the kit and kept refrigerated.

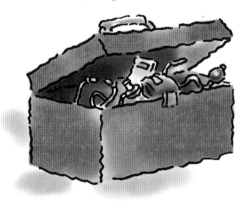

PACU *discharge criteria*

Typically, the patient must meet the following criteria before he can be discharged from the PACU:
- postanesthesia recovery score of 8 or above
- stable vital signs and oxygen saturation
- stable respiratory and cardiac status
- stable fluid balance status
- adequate pain control
- adequate control of nausea and vomiting
- surgical site that's free from complications, with a dry, intact dressing or minimal drainage and patent drainage tubes
- downward progression of the level of blockade from spinal anesthesia, with return of movement and sensation.

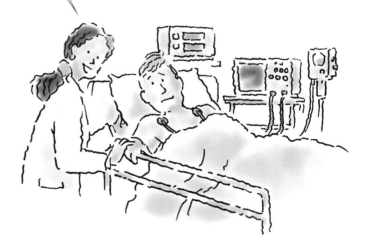

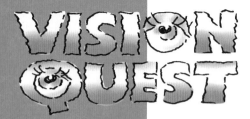

Able to label?

Label the parts of a PA catheter indicated here.

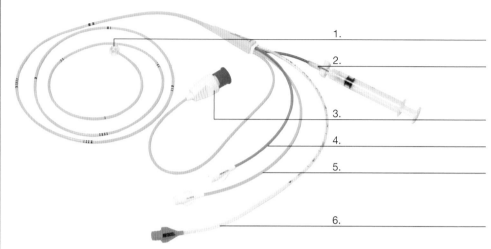

1. _____
2. _____
3. _____
4. _____
5. _____
6. _____

Matchmaker

Match each ECG rhythm strip with the corresponding arrhythmia.

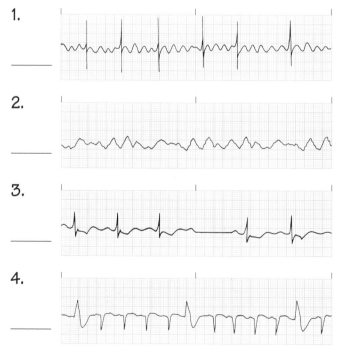

1. _____

2. _____

3. _____

4. _____

A. VF

B. Type II second-degree AV block

C. PVCs

D. Atrial flutter

6 Postoperative care

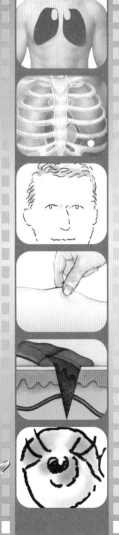

That's a wrap, folks! Remember that just as postproduction can make or break a movie, proper postoperative care of your patient ensures that he leaves the hospital healthy and ready to make his debut.

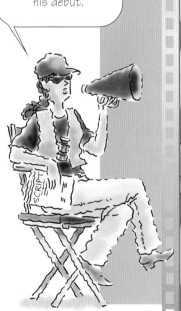

- Postoperative assessment 148
- Reducing the risk of complications 161
- Managing pain 166
- Managing postoperative complications 168
- Patient discharge needs 190
- Discharge summaries 192
- Vision quest 194

Remember to report any significant findings or changes immediately when caring for a postoperative patient.

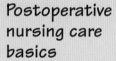

Postoperative assessment

Use a systematic approach to assessment. Compare your findings with intraoperative and preoperative findings, and report significant changes immediately.

Follow your facility's policy regarding frequency of assessment. Some protocols require assessment every 15 minutes until the patient stabilizes, every hour for the next 4 hours, and then every 4 hours.

Postoperative nursing care basics

The postoperative period extends from the time the patient leaves the operating room to his last follow-up visit with the surgeon. During recovery from anesthesia, he's monitored in the post-anesthesia care unit (PACU).

Next, the patient is transferred to the short-procedures, critical care, or medical-surgical unit. Nursing responsibilities in those units include:
■ confirming the patient's identity
■ positioning the patient in bed
■ assessing the operative site and drains
■ checking the I.V. site and I.V. flow rate
■ obtaining vital signs and oxygen saturation value
■ assessing the patient's pain level and comparing it to preoperative, intraoperative, and PACU levels
■ reporting significant findings.

Respiratory assessment

Assess the patient for:
■ airway patency and the need for an artificial airway
■ respiratory rate and depth
■ oxygen saturation and oxygen delivery system
■ breath sounds (noting adventitious sounds)
■ tracheal deviation from midline
■ chest symmetry, lung expansion, or accessory muscle use.

Anterior

Chest auscultation sequence

To distinguish between normal and adventitious breath sounds, press the stethoscope's diaphragm firmly against the patient's skin. Listen to a full inspiration and a full expiration at each site in the sequence shown. Remember to compare sound variations from one side to the other. Document adventitious sounds you hear, noting their locations.

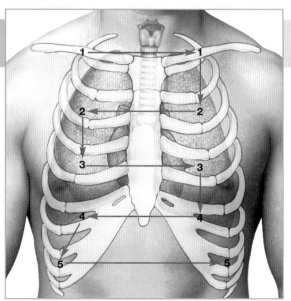

Qualities of normal breath sounds

Breath sound	Quality	Inspiration-expiration (I:E) ratio	Location	
Tracheal	Harsh, high-pitched	I = E	Above supraclavicular notch, over the trachea	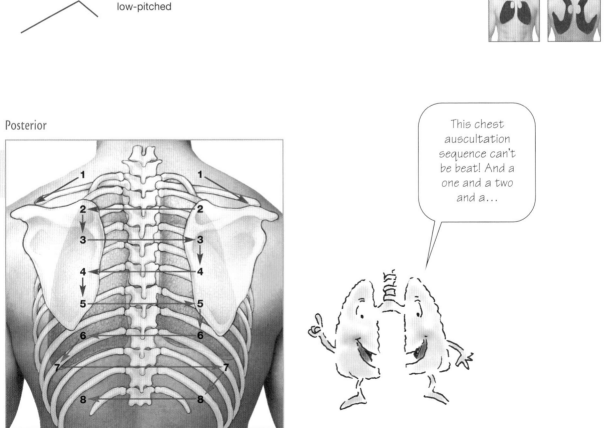
Bronchial	Loud, high-pitched	I < E	Just above clavicles on each side of the sternum, over the manubrium	
Bronchovesicular	Medium in loudness and pitch	I = E	Next to the sternum, between scapulae	
Vesicular	Soft, low-pitched	I > E	Remainder of lungs	

Posterior

This chest auscultation sequence can't be beat! And a one and a two and a...

Comparing adventitious breath sounds

Discontinuous sounds

Fine crackles
- Intermittent
- Nonmusical
- Soft (like hairs being rubbed together)
- High-pitched
- Short, cracking, popping sounds
- Heard during inspiration

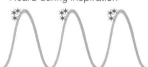

Coarse crackles
- Intermittent
- Nonmusical
- Loud
- Low-pitched
- Bubbling, gurgling sounds
- Heard during early inspiration and possibly during expiration

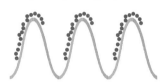

Adventitious breath sounds are never music to my ears. I prefer a nice aria any day.

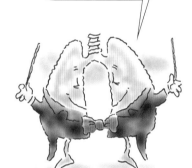

Continuous sounds

Wheezes
- Musical
- High-pitched
- Squeaky, whistling sounds
- Predominantly heard during expiration but may also occur during inspiration

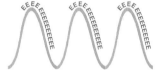

Rhonchi
- Musical
- Low-pitched
- Snoring, moaning sounds
- Heard during both inspiration and expiration but more prominent during expiration

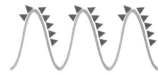

Cardiovascular assessment

Assess the patient's vital signs. Then assess for:
- ☐ S₁ and S₂ heart sounds (note additional sounds, such as S₃, S₄, or murmurs)
- ☐ amplitude and rhythm of peripheral pulses
- ☐ unilateral or bilateral leg edema.

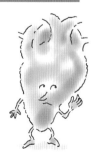

Heart sound sites

When auscultating heart sounds, place the stethoscope over the four sites illustrated here.

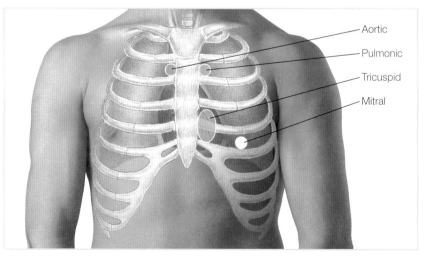

- Aortic
- Pulmonic
- Tricuspid
- Mitral

Neurologic assessment

Assess the patient for:
- level of consciousness (LOC)
- orientation
- ability to follow commands
- cranial nerve function
- motor function
- sensation
- reflexes.

Stages of altered arousal

1 Confusion
- Loss of the ability to think rapidly and clearly
- Impaired judgment and decision making

2 Disorientation
- Disorientation to time progressing to disorientation to place
- Impaired memory
- Lack of recognition of self (last)

3 Lethargy
- Limited spontaneous movement or speech
- Easy arousal with normal speech or touch
- Possible disorientation to time, place, or person

4 Obtundation
- Mild to moderate reduction in arousal
- Limited responsiveness to environment
- Ability to fall asleep easily without verbal or tactile stimulation
- Minimal response to questions

5 Stupor
- State of deep sleep or unresponsiveness
- Arousable with difficulty (motor or verbal response only to vigorous and repeated stimulation)
- Withdrawal or grabbing response to stimulation

6 Coma
- No motor or verbal response to external environment or any stimuli
- No response to noxious stimuli such as deep pain
- Not arousable by any stimulus

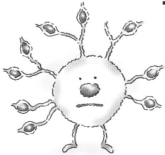

Picturing the cranial nerves

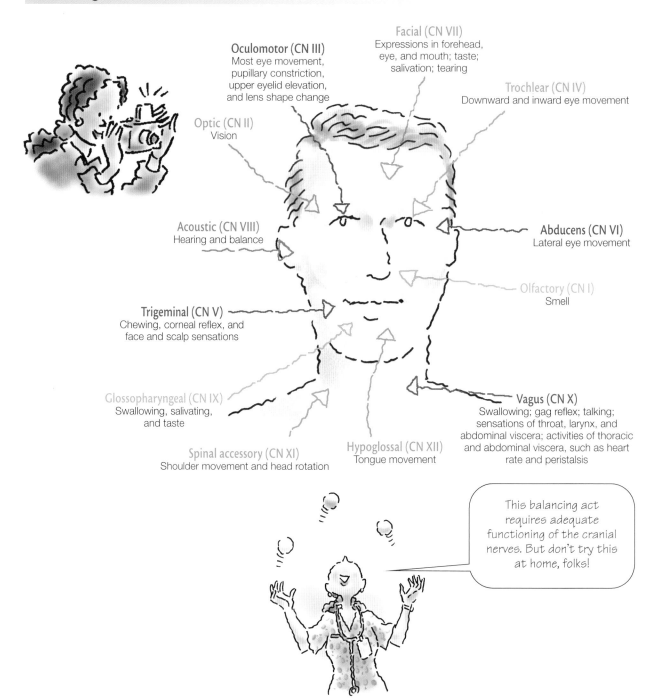

Oculomotor (CN III)
Most eye movement,
pupillary constriction,
upper eyelid elevation,
and lens shape change

Facial (CN VII)
Expressions in forehead,
eye, and mouth; taste;
salivation; tearing

Trochlear (CN IV)
Downward and inward eye movement

Optic (CN II)
Vision

Acoustic (CN VIII)
Hearing and balance

Abducens (CN VI)
Lateral eye movement

Olfactory (CN I)
Smell

Trigeminal (CN V)
Chewing, corneal reflex, and
face and scalp sensations

Glossopharyngeal (CN IX)
Swallowing, salivating,
and taste

Vagus (CN X)
Swallowing; gag reflex; talking;
sensations of throat, larynx, and
abdominal viscera; activities of thoracic
and abdominal viscera, such as heart
rate and peristalsis

Spinal accessory (CN XI)
Shoulder movement and head rotation

Hypoglossal (CN XII)
Tongue movement

This balancing act
requires adequate
functioning of the cranial
nerves. But don't try this
at home, folks!

Musculoskeletal assessment

Assess the patient for:
- proper body alignment
- symmetrical body parts
- active range of motion in all muscles and joints (note deficits or pain)
- equal bilateral muscle tone and strength.

Assessing leg strength

To ensure that the patient has adequate leg strength prior to ambulation, especially after spinal anesthesia or orthopedic or vascular surgery, ask him to lie in a supine position in bed and lift both legs. Note whether he lifts both legs at the same time and to the same distance. Then assess ankle strength by having the patient push his foot down against your resistance (plantar flexion) and then pull his foot up as you try to hold it down (dorsiflexion).

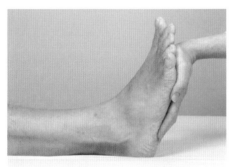

Plantar flexion

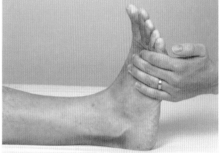

Dorsiflexion

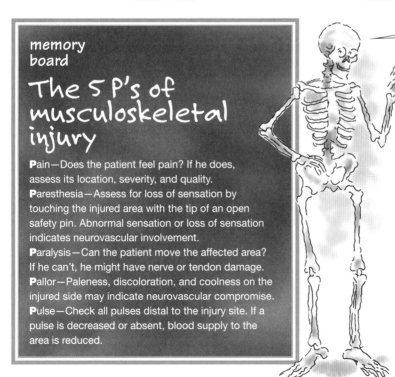

memory board

The 5 P's of musculoskeletal injury

Pain—Does the patient feel pain? If he does, assess its location, severity, and quality.

Paresthesia—Assess for loss of sensation by touching the injured area with the tip of an open safety pin. Abnormal sensation or loss of sensation indicates neurovascular involvement.

Paralysis—Can the patient move the affected area? If he can't, he might have nerve or tendon damage.

Pallor—Paleness, discoloration, and coolness on the injured side may indicate neurovascular compromise.

Pulse—Check all pulses distal to the injury site. If a pulse is decreased or absent, blood supply to the area is reduced.

When assessing a patient with a musculoskeletal injury, remember the 5 P's!

GI/GU assessment

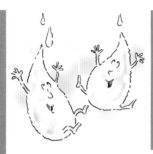

GI system

Assess the patient for:
- abdominal findings (such as softness, tenderness, or distention)
- bowel sounds
- nausea and vomiting
- type and amount of drainage from drainage tubes
- nasogastric (NG) tube patency.

GU system

Assess the patient for:
- fluid intake and output
- fluid and electrolyte balance
- type and amount of drainage from tubes and catheters
- thrills or bruits with an arteriovenous fistula.

All eyes on abdominal quadrants

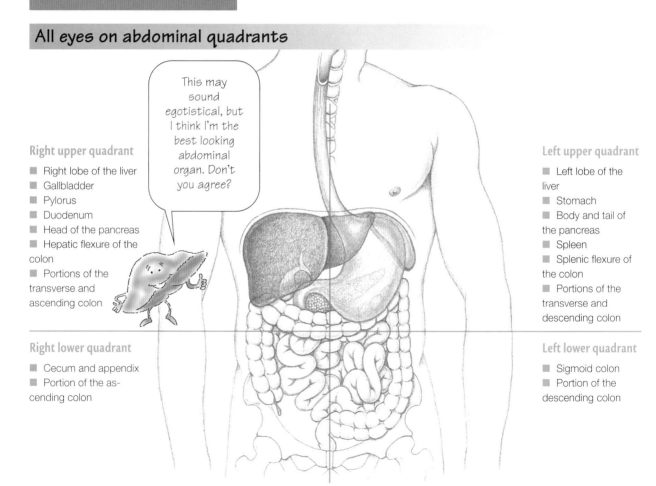

This may sound egotistical, but I think I'm the best looking abdominal organ. Don't you agree?

Right upper quadrant

- Right lobe of the liver
- Gallbladder
- Pylorus
- Duodenum
- Head of the pancreas
- Hepatic flexure of the colon
- Portions of the transverse and ascending colon

Left upper quadrant

- Left lobe of the liver
- Stomach
- Body and tail of the pancreas
- Spleen
- Splenic flexure of the colon
- Portions of the transverse and descending colon

Right lower quadrant

- Cecum and appendix
- Portion of the ascending colon

Left lower quadrant

- Sigmoid colon
- Portion of the descending colon

Integumentary assessment

Assess the patient for:
- skin texture and turgor
- skin temperature, moisture, and color
- risk of impaired skin integrity.

Assessing skin turgor in an adult

Gently squeeze the skin on the patient's forearm or sternal area between your thumb and forefinger, as shown.

If the patient's skin quickly returns to its original shape, it has normal turgor. If it returns to its original shape slowly over 30 seconds or maintains a tented position, as shown, it has poor turgor.

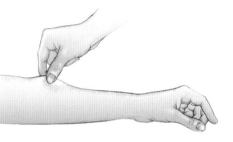

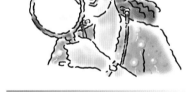

Cyanosis

Cyanosis (bluish discoloration of the skin and mucous membranes) may indicate poor cardiac output and tissue perfusion.

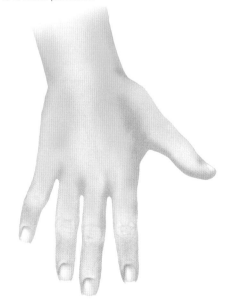

Pitting edema

When assessing skin texture and turgor, assess for edema, which may be pitting or nonpitting. To differentiate between the two, press your finger against a swollen area for 5 seconds, and then quickly remove it. With nonpitting edema, pressure leaves no indentation because fluid has coagulated in the tissues. Typically, the skin feels unusually tight and firm.

With pitting edema, pressure forces fluid into the underlying tissues, causing an indentation that slowly fills. To determine the severity of pitting edema, estimate the indentation's depth in centimeters: 1+, 2+, 3+, or 4+.

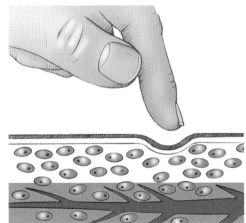

Surgical wound assessment

Assess the patient for:
- type of surgical wound closure
- location of drainage devices and type of wound drainage
- stage of wound healing.

Wound age

Typically, wounds are described as either acute or chronic.
- Acute wounds may be surgical or traumatic.
- Chronic wounds result from an underlying pathophysiologic disorder such as venous stasis.

Factors that affect wound healing

- Patient's age
- Nutritional status
- Oxygenation status
- General health
- Type of wound closure

Wound healing

A surgical wound may heal by:
- Primary intention—A surgical wound with an uncomplicated break in the skin and approximated edges; occurs in 4 to 14 days with minimal scarring
- Secondary intention—A wound left open because of significant tissue loss; takes longer for wound edges to come together, resulting in scarring and a higher complication rate
- Delayed primary closure—Wound edges are deliberately prevented from coming together for several days after surgery, resulting in more scarring than wounds healed by primary intention but less than those that heal by secondary intention.

Examining the surgical wound

When examining the surgical wound, be sure to follow the surgeon's orders. Don't remove the dressing without an order. Some dressings put pressure on the wound; others keep skin grafts intact.

If you note drainage stains on the dressing, estimate drainage quantity and note its color and odor. If the patient has a drainage device, record drainage amount and color. Make sure the device is secure and free from kinks. If the patient has an ileostomy or colostomy, describe its output.

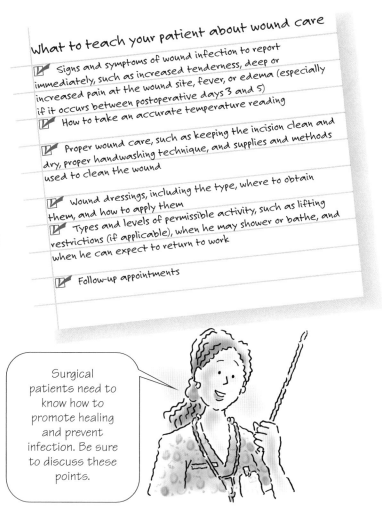

What to teach your patient about wound care

☑ Signs and symptoms of wound infection to report immediately, such as increased tenderness, deep or increased pain at the wound site, fever, or edema (especially if it occurs between postoperative days 3 and 5)

☑ How to take an accurate temperature reading

☑ Proper wound care, such as keeping the incision clean and dry, proper handwashing technique, and supplies and methods used to clean the wound

☑ Wound dressings, including the type, where to obtain them, and how to apply them

☑ Types and levels of permissible activity, such as lifting restrictions (if applicable), when he may shower or bathe, and when he can expect to return to work

☑ Follow-up appointments

Surgical patients need to know how to promote healing and prevent infection. Be sure to discuss these points.

> Ouch! The healing process begins at the instant of injury and proceeds through a repair "cascade" as described here.

How wounds heal

When tissue is damaged, serotonin, histamine, prostaglandins, and blood from the injured vessels fill the area. Blood platelets form a clot, and fibrin in the clot binds the wound edges together.

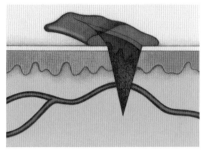

Lymphocytes initiate the inflammatory response, increasing capillary permeability. Wound edges swell; white blood cells from surrounding vessels move in and ingest bacteria and cellular debris, demolishing the clot. Redness, warmth, swelling, pain, and loss of function may occur.

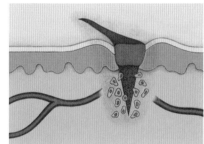

Adjacent healthy tissue supplies blood, nutrients, fibroblasts, proteins, and other building materials needed to form soft, pink, and highly vascular granulation tissue, which begins to bridge the area. Inflammation may decrease or signs and symptoms of infection (increased swelling and pain, fever, and pus-filled discharge) may develop.

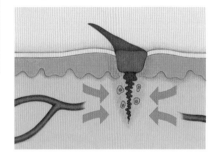

> Late in the repair process, a new layer of surface cells replaces the destroyed layer.

> That's right. I'm glad I've got you, babe!

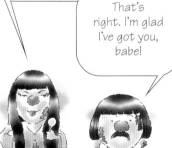

Fibroblasts in the granulation tissue secrete collagen, a gluelike substance. Collagen fibers crisscross the area, forming scar tissue. Meanwhile, epithelial cells at the wound edge multiply and migrate toward the wound center. A new layer of surface cells replaces the layer that was destroyed. New healthy tissue or granulation tissue (if blood supply is inadequate) appears.

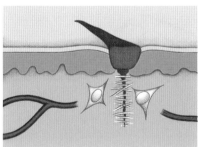

Damaged tissue (including lymphatics, blood vessels, and stromal matrices) regenerates. Collagen fibers shorten, and the scar diminishes in size. Scar size may decrease and normal function may return or the scar may hypertrophy, leading to keloid formation and contractures.

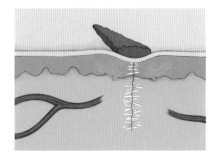

Suture materials and methods

Mattress continuous suture

Connected mattress stitches with a knot at the beginning and end.

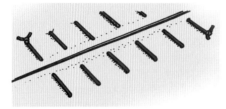

Plain continuous suture

Connected stitches with the thread knotted at the beginning and end of the suture. (Also called a *continuous running suture.*)

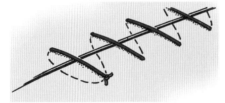

Blanket continuous suture

Looped stitches with a knot at the beginning and end.

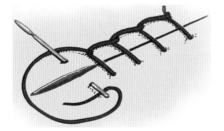

Suture materials

Nonabsorbable sutures:
- are used to close the skin surface
- provide strength and immobility
- cause minimal tissue irritation
- are made of silk, cotton, stainless steel, or Dacron.

Absorbable sutures:
- are used when suture removal is undesirable
- are made of:
  - chromic catgut—a natural catgut treated with chromium trioxide to improve strength and prolong absorption time
  - plain catgut—a material that's absorbed faster and is more likely to cause irritation than chromic catgut
  - synthetic materials (such as polyglycolic acid)—materials that are replacing catgut because they're stronger, more durable, and less irritating.

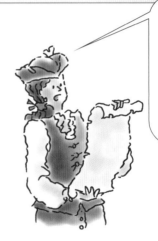

Hear ye, hear ye! The materials used to close surgical wounds vary with the suturing method.

Mattress interrupted suture

Independent stitches with both threads crossing beneath the suture line, leaving only a small portion of suture exposed on each side of the wound.

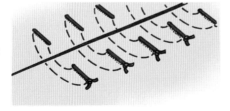

Plain interrupted suture

Individual sutures sewn with a separate piece of thread. Half the thread length crosses under the suture line and the other half crosses above the skin surface.

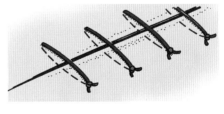

Types of adhesive skin closures

Steri-Strips

Steri-Strips (thin strips of sterile, nonwoven tape) are a primary means of holding a wound closed after suture removal.

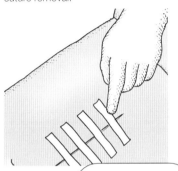

Butterfly closures

Butterfly closures have two sterile, waterproof adhesive strips linked by a narrow, nonadhesive "bridge." They're used to hold small wounds closed to promote healing after suture removal.

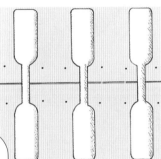

> The two most common types of adhesive skin closures are Steri-Strips and butterfly closures.

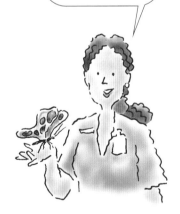

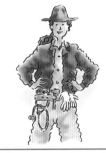

Come equipped

Using a closed-wound drainage system

The portable closed-wound drainage system draws drainage from a wound site, such as the chest wall postmastectomy (shown below top), by means of a Y tube. To empty the drainage, remove the plug and empty it into a graduated cylinder. To reestablish suction, compress the drainage unit against a firm surface to expel air and, while holding it down, replace the plug with your other hand (as shown below right). The same principle applies to the Jackson-Pratt bulb drain (shown below left).

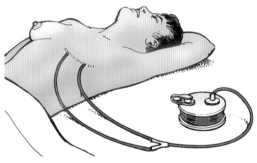

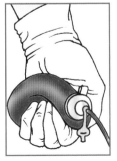

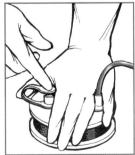

Pain assessment

The Joint Commission on Accreditation of Healthcare Organizations (JCAHO) requires that patients be asked on admission if they're experiencing pain. Patients who report pain must be assessed further by licensed personnel using a standard pain screening tool.

If your facility is JCAHO accredited, check its policies and procedures to determine how often to assess the patient's pain, which screening tool to use, and which reported pain level warrants further assessment and action.

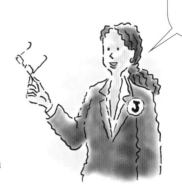

Assess the patient's pain using your facility's approved scale. In many facilities, a pain level of 4 or higher on a 0-to-10 scale warrants further assessment and action.

memory board

Use the PQRST mnemonic device to obtain more information about your patient's pain. Asking the questions below elicits important details.

Provocative or palliative

- What provokes or worsens your pain?
- What relieves or causes the pain to subside?

Quality or quantity

- What does the pain feel like? Is it aching, intense, knifelike, burning, or cramping?
- Are you having pain right now? If so, is it more or less severe than usual?
- To what degree does the pain affect your normal activities?
- Do you have other symptoms along with pain, such as nausea or vomiting?

Region and radiation

- Where's your pain?
- Does the pain radiate to other parts of your body?

Severity

- How severe is your pain? How would you rate it on a 0-to-10 scale, with 0 being no pain and 10 being the worst pain imaginable?
- How would you describe the intensity of your pain at its best? At its worst? Right now?

Timing

- When did your pain begin?
- At what time of day is your pain best? What time is it worst?
- Is the onset sudden or gradual?
- Is the pain constant or intermittent?

Reducing the risk of complications

To reduce your patient's risk for postoperative complications, be sure to turn and reposition him as needed, encourage deep breathing and coughing, monitor his nutritional status and fluid balance, and promote exercise and ambulation.

Turning and repositioning the patient

To promote circulation and reduce the risk of skin breakdown, turn and reposition the patient every 2 hours. Be aware that after some neurologic or musculoskeletal surgery, turning and repositioning may be contraindicated. Be sure to follow postoperative orders.

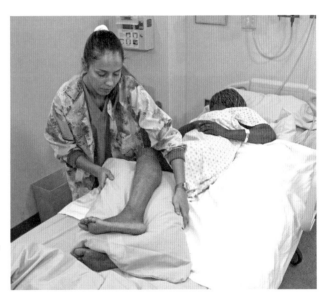

Repositioning the patient

Although your patient won't be ready to turn cartwheels like this right after surgery, you should turn and reposition him regularly, if indicated.

Encouraging deep breathing and coughing

Deep breathing promotes lung expansion, which in turn helps clear anesthetics from the body. Along with coughing, deep breathing also helps prevent hypostatic pneumonia caused by secretion buildup in the airways. Encourage coughing exercises unless your patient is recovering from neurosurgery or eye surgery for which coughing is contraindicated.

> Taking a deep breath increases lung volume, boosts alveolar inflation, promotes venous return, and loosens respiratory secretions.

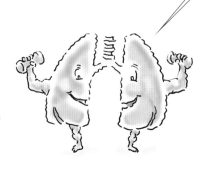

Come equipped

Using incentive spirometry

An incentive spirometer is a breathing device that helps the patient achieve maximal ventilation by encouraging him to take a deep breath and hold it for several seconds. It measures inspiratory effort (flow rate) in cubic centimeters per second.

> Encourage the patient to deep breathe and cough every hour while awake. Also teach him how to use an incentive spirometer.

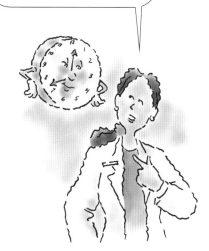

Volume incentive spirometer

The volume incentive spirometer is activated when the patient inhales a certain volume of air. By estimating the volume of air inhaled, it measures lung inflation more precisely. It's used with patients at high risk for atelectasis.

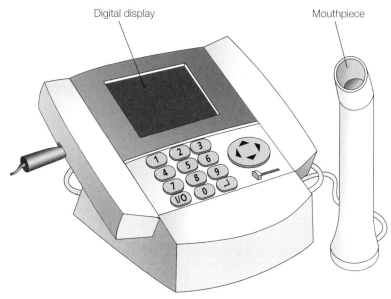

Digital display

Mouthpiece

■ Help the patient into a comfortable sitting or semi-Fowler's position to promote optimal lung expansion. If you're using a flow incentive spirometer and the patient can't assume or maintain this position, tell him he can use the spirometer in any position, as long as it remains upright. (Tilting it decreases the required patient effort and makes the exercise less effective.)

■ Instruct the patient to exhale normally, insert the mouthpiece, and close his lips tightly around it. (A weak seal may alter flow or volume readings.)

■ Tell the patient to inhale as slowly and deeply as possible. If he has trouble doing this, advise him to suck as he would through a straw but more slowly. Instruct him to retain the entire volume of in-haled air for 3 seconds or, if the device has a light indicator, until the light shuts off. This deep breath (called a *sustained maximal inspiration*) creates sustained transpulmonary pressure near the end of inspiration.

■ Instruct the patient to remove the mouthpiece and exhale normally. Let him relax and take several normal breaths before attempting another breath with the spirometer. Have him repeat this sequence 5 to 10 times during waking hours. Note tidal volumes.

■ Evaluate the patient's ability to cough effectively, and encourage him to cough after each effort to help loosen secretions and promote their removal. Observe expectorated secretions.

Flow incentive spirometer

The flow incentive spirometer contains plastic floats, which rise according to how much air the patient pulls through the device during inhalation. It's used with patients at low risk for atelectasis.

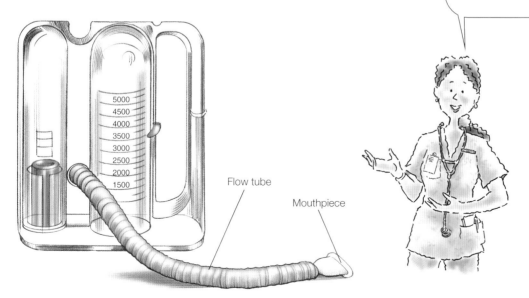

5000
4500
4000
3500
3000
2500
2000
1500

Flow tube

Mouthpiece

Remember to auscultate the patient's lungs after incentive spirometry and compare your findings with your baseline assessment.

Monitoring nutrition and fluid balance

Adequate nutritional and fluid intake is essential for promoting healing, ensuring proper hydration, and providing energy to meet the increased basal metabolism associated with surgery. If the patient had a protein deficiency, was immunocompromised before surgery, or had extensive surgery to the GI tract, expect to deliver supplemental protein by parenteral nutrition during the postoperative period.

Use an intake and output flow sheet to record your patient's fluid intake and output. When documenting input, be sure to include:
- ice chips and oral fluids
- I.V. fluids
- tube feedings
- blood products
- irrigation fluid.

When documenting output, be sure to:
- include urine, tube drainage, and wound drainage
- note its source (quantity, color, consistency, and duration)
- notify the surgeon of significant changes (such as changes in the color or consistency of NG contents from dark green to a coffee-ground texture, or an unexpectedly large output).

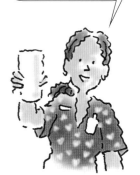

Be sure to measure your patient's fluid intake and output.

Intake and output record

Name: __Josephine Klein__

Medical record #: __49731__

Admission date: __2/13/06__

	Intake					Output				
	Oral	Tube feeding	Instilled	I.V.	**Total**	Urine	Emesis	NG tube	Other	**Total**
Date 2/15/06										
0700-1500	250	320	H₂0 50	1100	1720	1355				1355
1500-2300	200	320	H₂0 50	1100	1670	1200				1200
2300-0700	0	320	H₂0 50	1100	1470	1500				1500
24 hour total	450	960	H₂0 150	3300	4860	4055				4055

Promoting exercise and ambulation

Early postoperative exercise and ambulation can significantly reduce the risk of thromboembolism and improve ventilation. To prevent joint contractures and muscle atrophy and to promote circulation, perform passive range-of-motion (ROM) exercises. Better yet, encourage the patient to perform active ROM exercises. As he performs them, you can assess his strength and tolerance for activity.

Before encouraging ambulation, have the patient dangle his legs over the side of the bed and perform deep-breathing exercises. His tolerance for these activities helps predict his tolerance for being out of bed.

Teaching about active ROM exercises

Leg and knee exercises

1 Lie on your bed. Bend one leg so your knee is straight up and your foot is flat on the bed.
2 Raise your foot, bend the other leg, and slowly bring your knee as far toward your chest as you can without discomfort.
3 Straighten this leg slowly while you lower it.
4 Repeat this exercise with your other leg.

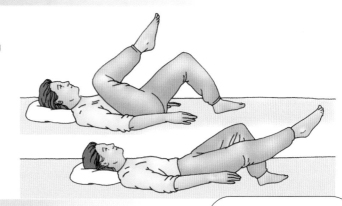

Ankle and foot exercises

1 Raise one foot and point your toes away from you. Move this foot in a circular motion—first to the right, then to the left.
2 Point your toes back toward you. With your foot in this position, make a circle with it—first to the right, then to the left.
3 Now do the same exercise with your other foot.

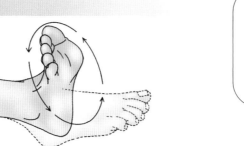

Don't forget to document your patient's frequency of movement, tolerance for ambulation, and analgesic use.

Toe exercises

1 Sit in a chair or lie on your bed. Stretch your legs out in front of you, with your heels resting on the floor or the bed. Slowly bend your toes down and away from you.
2 Bend your toes up and back toward you.
3 Spread out your toes so they're totally separated. Then squeeze your toes together.

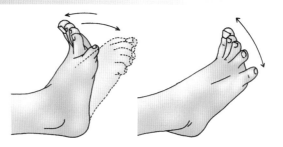

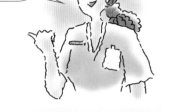

Teach the postoperative patient the following techniques to reduce pain when he moves, coughs, or breathes deeply.

Managing pain

Always monitor and promote your patient's comfort postoperatively. Administer analgesics, as ordered, and teach him techniques to reduce incisional pain. Pain management may also involve epidural analgesia or patient-controlled analgesia (PCA).

Promoting comfort

A postoperative patient may be unable to find a comfortable position. As needed, use physical measures, such as positioning, back rubs, and environmental modifications, to promote comfort and enhance analgesic drug effectiveness.

Administering analgesics

Analgesics commonly used during the postoperative period include opioids, nonopioid analgesics, and adjuvant analgesics (such as anticonvulsants).

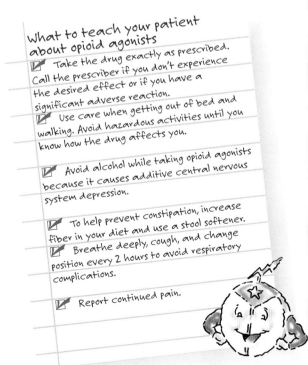

What to teach your patient about opioid agonists

☑ Take the drug exactly as prescribed. Call the prescriber if you don't experience the desired effect or if you have a significant adverse reaction.

☑ Use care when getting out of bed and walking. Avoid hazardous activities until you know how the drug affects you.

☑ Avoid alcohol while taking opioid agonists because it causes additive central nervous system depression.

☑ To help prevent constipation, increase fiber in your diet and use a stool softener.

☑ Breathe deeply, cough, and change position every 2 hours to avoid respiratory complications.

☑ Report continued pain.

Tips for reducing incisional pain

Proper movement

Instruct the patient to:
- use the bed's side rails for support when he moves and turns
- move slowly and smoothly, without sudden jerks
- delay moving until after his pain medication has taken effect, if possible
- frequently move parts of his body not affected by surgery so they won't become stiff and sore
- make sure he's medicated so he can move comfortably
- ask a staff member to help if moving alone is difficult.

Splinting the incision

After chest or abdominal surgery, splinting the incision may help the patient reduce pain when he coughs or moves.

Splinting with the hands

Instruct the patient to place one hand above and the other hand below his incision (as shown), and then press gently and breathe normally when he moves.

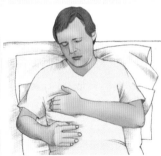

Splinting with a pillow

Alternatively, the patient may place a small pillow over his incision. As he holds the pillow in place with his hands and arms, he should press gently (as shown), breathe normally, and move to a sitting or standing position.

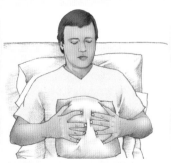

Epidural anesthesia

Usually initiated in the PACU, epidural analgesia provides effective pain management, promotes early ambulation, and speeds recovery and adequate respiratory function. Typically, nurses with special training manage patient care.

PCA

An effective measure to control acute postoperative pain, PCA allows the patient to self-administer analgesic doses while providing optimal opioid dosing and maintaining a constant serum drug level.

> Abracadabra — the pain goes away! Pain relief is a magical feeling for many patients.

Come equipped

Understanding PCA

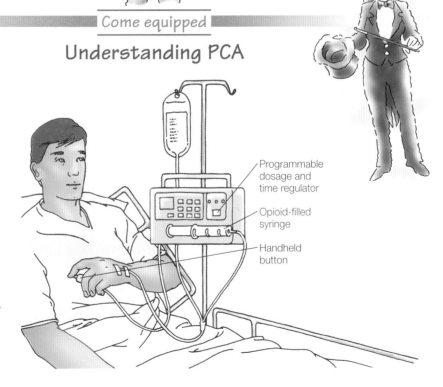

A PCA system consists of a syringe injection pump piggybacked into an I.V. or subcutaneous infusion port. When the patient presses a button, he receives a preset bolus dose of medication. To prevent overdose, the surgeon orders the bolus dose and the "lock-out" time between boluses. The device automatically records the number of times that the patient presses the button, helping the surgeon adjust the dosage.

In some cases, the PCA system allows a dosage reduction—perhaps because the patient feels more control over pain relief and knows analgesia is available quickly when he needs it. This tends to reduce stress and anxiety, which can exacerbate pain.

Programmable dosage and time regulator

Opioid-filled syringe

Handheld button

Managing postoperative complications

Common postoperative complications include atelectasis and pneumonia, compartment syndrome, fat embolism, hypovolemia, paralytic ileus, pericarditis, pressure ulcers, pulmonary embolism, septicemia and septic shock, thrombophlebitis, urine retention, wound dehiscence and evisceration, and wound infection.

Atelectasis

Hypoventilation and excessive retained secretions may lead to atelectasis (lung tissue collapse).

What to look for

- Diminished or absent breath sounds over the affected area
- Dullness on percussion
- With massive collapse, reduced chest expansion; mediastinal shift toward the collapsed side; fever; restlessness; confusion; worsening dyspnea; and increased blood pressure, pulse rate, and respiratory rates

What to do

- Encourage the patient to perform deep-breathing and coughing exercises every hour when awake.
- Demonstrate how to use an incentive spirometer.
- Perform chest physiotherapy and administer humidified air or oxygen.
- Reposition the patient every 2 hours and elevate the head of the bed.

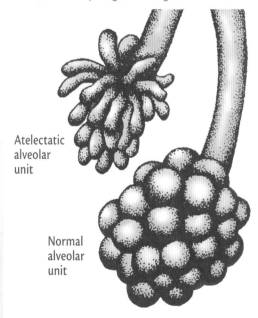

Postop pitfall

Atelectasis

Normally, air-filled alveoli exchange oxygen and carbon dioxide with capillary blood. In atelectasis, airless, shrunken alveoli can't accomplish gas exchange.

Atelectatic alveolar unit

Normal alveolar unit

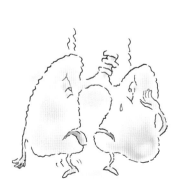

Pneumonia

Atelectasis provides a medium for bacterial growth and may set the stage for stasis pneumonia.

What to look for

■ Sudden onset of shaking chills, with high fever and headache
■ Dyspnea, tachypnea, sharp chest pain exacerbated by inspiration
■ Productive cough with pinkish or rust-colored sputum
■ Diminished breath sounds or crackles over the affected lung area
■ Cyanosis with hypoxemia confirmed by arterial blood gas measurement
■ Patchy infiltrates or areas of consolidation on chest X-ray

What to do

■ Maintain a patent airway and adequate oxygenation.
■ Administer supplemental oxygen.
■ Give analgesics to relieve pleuritic chest pain.
■ Obtain sputum cultures.
■ Give antibiotics.
■ Provide adequate fluids and a high-calorie diet.
■ Encourage the patient to perform deep-breathing and coughing exercises every hour when awake.
■ Demonstrate how to use an incentive spirometer.
■ Reposition the patient every 2 hours and elevate the head of the bed.

Types of pneumonia

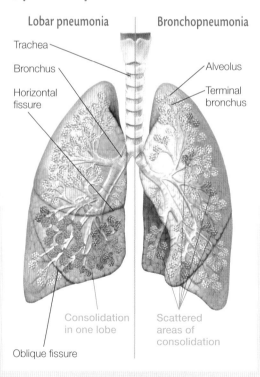

Lobar pneumonia

Bronchopneumonia

Trachea

Bronchus

Horizontal fissure

Alveolus

Terminal bronchus

Consolidation in one lobe

Scattered areas of consolidation

Oblique fissure

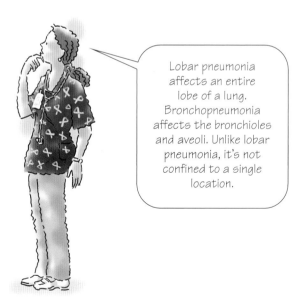

Lobar pneumonia affects an entire lobe of a lung. Bronchopneumonia affects the bronchioles and aveoli. Unlike lobar pneumonia, it's not confined to a single location.

Compartment syndrome

Compartment syndrome occurs when edema or bleeding increases pressure within a muscle compartment to the point of impeding circulation to muscles and nerves within the compartment. A limb-threatening condition requiring immediate intervention, it's most common in the lower arm, hand, lower leg, or foot.

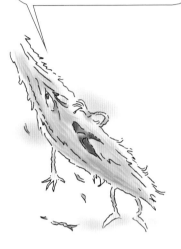

Compartment syndrome causes pain that doesn't improve with analgesia or elevation of the extremity.

What to look for

■ Intense, deep, throbbing pain that's out of proportion to the injury and doesn't improve with analgesia
■ Numbness and tingling distal to the affected muscle
■ Absent peripheral pulses in the affected extremity
■ Pallor or mottling of the affected area
■ Decreased movement, muscle strength, and sensation in the affected extremity

What to do

■ Position the affected extremity at heart level.
■ Remove constricting clothing and dressings.
■ Administer analgesics.
■ Assess the affected extremity regularly, performing neurovascular checks to detect signs of impaired circulation and nerve function.
■ Prepare the patient for an intracompartmental pressure check and Doppler ultrasound.
■ If indicated, prepare the patient for an emergency fasciotomy.

Be sure to monitor your patient for compartment syndrome. Keep these risk factors in mind.

Risks for compartment syndrome

■ Constrictive casts and dressings
■ Long bone fractures
■ Orthopedic surgery
■ Crush injuries
■ Thermal injuries

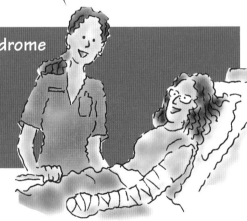

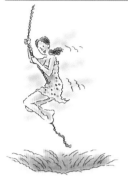

Postop pitfall
What happens in compartment syndrome

These illustrations show a cross-section of a normal calf and a cross-section of a calf with compartment syndrome. The illustration on the right shows how a fasciotomy can relieve increased pressure in the extremity by allowing muscle tissue to expand outward. In the procedure, the surgeon makes two long incisions in the fascia down the affected extremity. Typically, these wounds are closed in a second surgical procedure 2 to 3 days later.

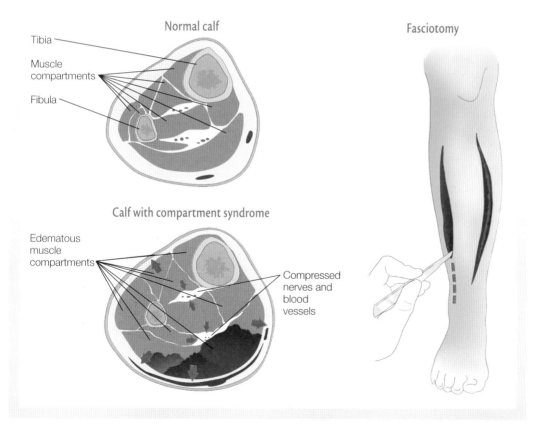

Normal calf

Tibia

Muscle compartments

Fibula

Calf with compartment syndrome

Edematous muscle compartments

Compressed nerves and blood vessels

Fasciotomy

Fat embolism

Posttraumatic fat embolization may occur as bone marrow releases fat into the veins. If the fat particle lodges in the lungs, it could obstruct the pulmonary vascular bed. If it passes into the arteries, it eventually could disturb the respiratory and circulatory systems.

Fat embolism typically occurs 12 to 48 hours after an injury. Although most commonly seen as a complication of long bone fracture, it may also follow severe soft-tissue bruising or fatty liver injury.

What to look for

- Tachycardia
- Fever
- Altered LOC (possibly coma)
- Anxiety and restlessness
- Blood-tinged sputum
- Cyanosis
- Petechial rash over the anterior chest, neck, shoulders, and axillae and buccal membranes
- Seizures

What to do

- Monitor vital signs, hemodynamic status, and oxygen saturation.
- Assess heart and breath sounds.
- Administer prescribed drugs, such as corticosteroids and heparin, and oxygen.
- Assist with endotracheal (ET) intubation and ventilation.
- Assess the patient's LOC regularly.
- Prepare the patient for diagnostic tests, such as arterial blood gas analysis, computed tomography, and chest X-ray.
- Keep the affected limb immobilized and properly aligned.

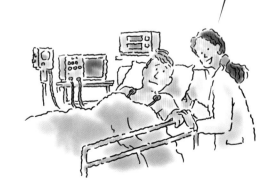

If your patient has a fat embolism, promote rest and relaxation and provide emotional support.

Postop pitfall

How fat embolism threatens pulmonary circulation

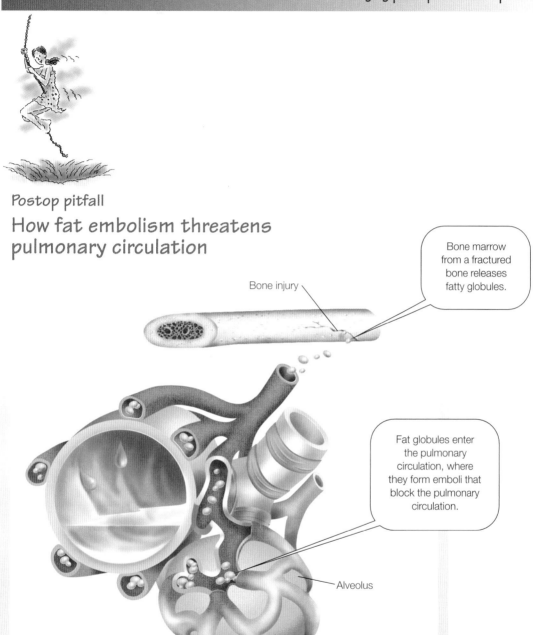

Hypovolemia

Hypovolemia (total blood volume loss of 15% to 25%) may result from:

- blood loss at the surgical site
- severe dehydration
- third-space fluid sequestration (as in burns, peritonitis, intestinal obstruction, or acute pancreatitis)
- fluid loss from excessive vomiting or diarrhea.

Untreated, hypovolemia leads to hypovolemic shock.

What to look for

- Lethargy
- Hypotension
- Rapid, weak pulse
- Cool, clammy and, possibly, mottled skin
- Rapid, shallow respirations
- Oliguria or anuria

What to do

- Provide supplemental oxygen to increase oxygenation.
- Prepare the patient for ET intubation.
- Administer an I.V. crystalloid solution, such as normal saline, to increase blood pressure.
- Administer a colloid, such as plasma, albumin, or dextran, to restore urine output and fluid volume.
- Administer packed red cells to restore blood volume.
- If fluid resuscitation is unsuccessful, give vasopressors to improve perfusion and maintain blood pressure.

Postop pitfall

Understanding hypovolemic shock

Internal or external fluid loss
Decreased intravascular fluid volume
Diminished venous return
Reduced preload (filling pressure)
Decreased stroke volume
Decreased cardiac output
Reduced mean arterial blood pressure
Decreased tissue perfusion
Reduced oxygen and nutrient delivery to cells
Multiple organ dysfunction syndrome

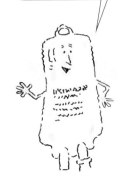

If your patient has hypovolemia, expect to give an I.V. crystalloid solution, such as normal saline or lactated Ringer's, to increase blood pressure.

Paralytic ileus

For the first 24 to 72 hours after surgery, the patient may have sluggish peristalsis and paralytic ileus, causing abdominal distention. Paralytic ileus occurs when autonomic GI tract innervation is disrupted from intraoperative intestinal manipulation, hypokalemia, wound infection, or use of codeine, morphine, or atropine.

What to look for

■ Severe abdominal distention, possibly with vomiting
■ Decreased or absent bowel sounds
■ Severe constipation or passage of flatus and small, liquid stools

What to do

■ Encourage ambulation.
■ Withhold food and fluids.
■ Insert an NG tube.
■ Monitor for nausea and vomiting, and give an antiemetic.

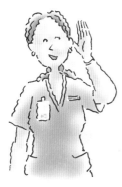

Interpreting abnormal abdominal sounds

Sound and description	Location	Possible causes
Abnormal bowel sounds		
Hyperactive sounds (unrelated to hunger)	Any quadrant	Diarrhea, laxative use, or early intestinal obstruction
Hypoactive, then absent, sounds	Any quadrant	Paralytic ileus or peritonitis
High-pitched tinkling sounds	Any quadrant	Intestinal fluid and air under tension in a dilated bowel
High-pitched rushing sounds accompanied by abdominal cramps	Any quadrant	Intestinal obstruction
Systolic bruits		
Vascular blowing sounds	Over abdominal aorta	Partial arterial obstruction or turbulent blood flow
	Over renal artery	Renal artery stenosis
	Over iliac artery	Iliac artery stenosis
Venous hum		
Continuous, medium-pitched tone created by blood flow in a large, engorged vascular organ	Epigastric and umbilical regions	Increased collateral circulation between portal and systemic venous systems (as in cirrhosis)
Friction rub		
Harsh, grating sound	Over liver and spleen	Inflammation of the peritoneal surface of liver

If you hear a harsh, grating sound over the liver and spleen, suspect inflammation of the liver's peritoneal surface.

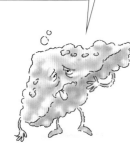

Pericarditis

Pericarditis is an acute or chronic inflammation of the pericardium (fibroserous sac that envelops, supports, and protects the heart). Postoperatively, pericarditis may arise from bacterial, fungal, or viral infection or from postcardiac injury that leaves the pericardium intact but causes blood to leak into the pericardial cavity.

What to look for

■ Sharp, sudden pain that starts over the sternum and radiates to the neck, shoulders, back, and arms
■ Pericardial pain and pericardial friction rub. (To distinguish pericardial pain from pain caused by myocardial ischemia, assess the patient's pain relative to deep inspiration and body position. Pericardial pain worsens with deep inspiration and subsides when the patient sits up and leans forward.)
■ Fever

What to do

■ Keep the patient on complete bed rest as long as fever persists.
■ Provide an analgesic and oxygen.
■ Monitor for signs of cardiac compression or tamponade, such as decreased blood pressure, increased central venous pressure, and paradoxical pulse.
■ Prepare the patient for pericardectomy, if indicated.

Assessing for pericardial friction rub

If you suspect that your patient has a pericardial friction rub, first have him sit up and lean forward to bring his heart closer to his chest. Then auscultate using the diaphragm of the stethoscope. A pericardial friction rub has a high pitch and a grating or scratchy quality.

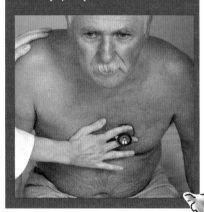

A patient with a pericardial friction rub experiences less pain when sitting up and leaning forward.

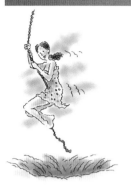

Postop pitfall
Tissue changes in pericarditis

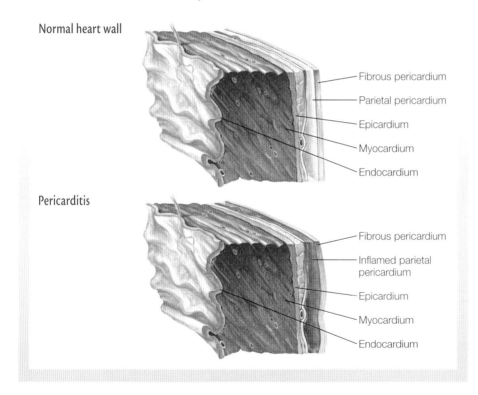

Normal heart wall

- Fibrous pericardium
- Parietal pericardium
- Epicardium
- Myocardium
- Endocardium

Pericarditis

- Fibrous pericardium
- Inflamed parietal pericardium
- Epicardium
- Myocardium
- Endocardium

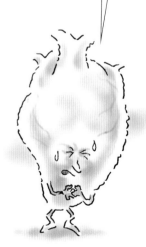

Ouch! Pericarditis causes sharp, sudden pain, not to mention fever. I think I need to go to bed and stay there for awhile.

Pressure ulcers

Pressure ulcers result from prolonged pressure against the skin, which impairs circulation to the affected area and deprives tissues of oxygen and other nutrients. Risk factors include:
- advanced age
- immobility
- incontinence
- infection
- hypotension
- poor nutrition
- decreased albumin levels.

What to look for

- Reddened skin
- Blanching erythema with finger compression (may indicate a pressure ulcer developing over a bony prominence)
- Nonblanchable erythema (suggesting the onset of tissue destruction)

What to do

- Assess the ulcer's location and stage. Note its length, width, and depth (in centimeters).
- Inspect for drainage, necrotic tissue, granulation tissue, and epithelialization.
- Protect the ulcer from further injury.
- Provide adequate nutrition to promote wound healing.
- Provide an optimal wound-healing environment by using appropriate dressings to keep moist tissue moist and dry tissue dry.
- Prepare the patient for debridement of necrotic tissue, if indicated.

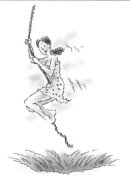

Postop pitfall

Staging pressure ulcers

You can use pressure ulcer characteristics gained from your assessment to stage the pressure ulcer, as described here. The most widely used system for staging pressure ulcers is the classification system developed by the National Pressure Ulcer Advisory Panel. Staging reflects the anatomic depth of exposed tissue. Keep in mind that if the wound contains necrotic tissue, you won't be able to determine the stage until you can see the wound base.

Stage 1

An area of skin that develops observable, pressure-related changes that include persistent redness in patients with light skin or persistent red, blue, or purple color in patients with darker skin. Other indicators include pain, itching, warmth, edema, or hardness at the site.

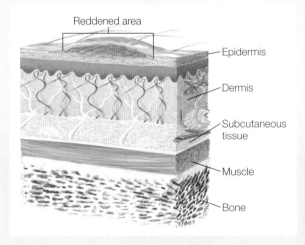

Reddened area
Epidermis
Dermis
Subcutaneous tissue
Muscle
Bone

Stage 2

Superficial partial-thickness wound that presents clinically as an abrasion, blister, or shallow crater involving the epidermis, dermis, or both.

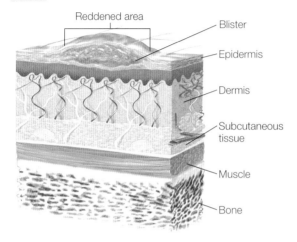

Labels: Reddened area, Blister, Epidermis, Dermis, Subcutaneous tissue, Muscle, Bone

Stage 4

Full-thickness wound with extensive damage, tissue necrosis, or damage to muscle, bone, or structures, such as joints and tendons. The wound may undermine to neighboring tissues and develop sinus tracts.

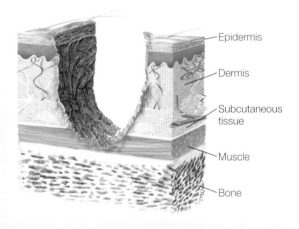

Labels: Epidermis, Dermis, Subcutaneous tissue, Muscle, Bone

Stage 3

Full-thickness wound with tissue damage or necrosis of subcutaneous tissue that can extend down to, but not through, underlying fasciae. The wound presents clinically as a deep crater that may undermine to neighboring tissue.

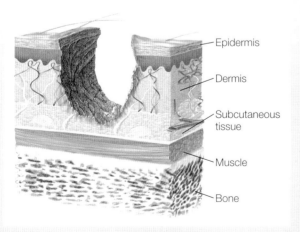

Labels: Epidermis, Dermis, Subcutaneous tissue, Muscle, Bone

Pulmonary embolism

Pulmonary embolism is an obstruction of the pulmonary arterial bed. It occurs when foreign matter, such as a blood clot that has broken away from a vein, obstructs a pulmonary artery branch. During the postoperative period, immobility and venous stasis increase the risk for pumonary embolism.

What to look for

- Dyspnea
- Rapid, shallow respirations
- Sudden anginal or pleuritic chest pain
- Fine to coarse crackles over the affected lung area
- Possible cyanosis or blood-tinged sputum
- Restlessness
- Low-grade fever
- Tachycardia
- Thready pulse
- Hypotension

What to do

- Administer oxygen.
- Prepare the patient for ET intubation and mechanical ventilation.
- Place the patient in a comfortable position, with the head of the bed elevated.
- Initiate cardiac monitoring and watch for arrhythmias.
- Give drugs, such as heparin, to inhibit new thrombus formation and fibrinolytics to enhance fibrinolysis of pulmonary emboli.
- Administer vasopressors to treat hypotension.
- Prepare the patient for insertion of a vena cava filter or surgical embolectomy, if necessary.

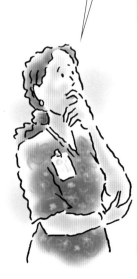

After surgery, immobility and venous stasis can cause pulmonary embolism.

Understanding pulmonary embolism

Blood clot forms in the deep venous system.

⬇

Clot dislodges and travels through the systemic venous system, right chambers of heart, and into the pulmonary circulation.

⬇

Clot lodges in branch of the circulatory system.

⬇

Blood flow distal to the obstruction is blocked.

⬇

Embolus prevents alveoli from producing enough surfactant to maintain alveolar integrity; alveoli collapse and atelectasis develops.

⬇

A large clot can cause tissue death.

> Here you see multiple emboli lodged in the small branches of the left pulmonary artery.

Postop pitfall
Pulmonary emboli

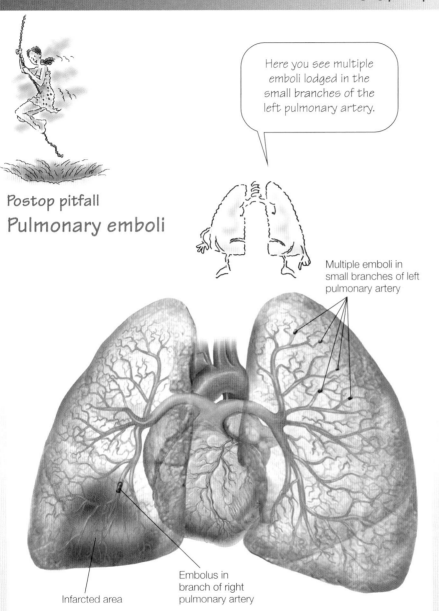

Multiple emboli in small branches of left pulmonary artery

Embolus in branch of right pulmonary artery

Infarcted area

Septicemia

A systemic infection of the bloodstream, septicemia may stem from a break in aseptic technique during surgery or wound care or from peritonitis (as from a ruptured appendix or an ectopic pregnancy). Postoperatively, the most common cause of septicemia is *Escherichia coli* infection.

What to look for

- Fever
- Chills
- Rash
- Abdominal distention
- Prostration
- Pain
- Headache
- Nausea and diarrhea

What to do

- Obtain a urine specimen, blood samples, and wound specimens for culture and sensitivity tests.
- Administer antibiotics.
- Monitor vital signs and LOC.

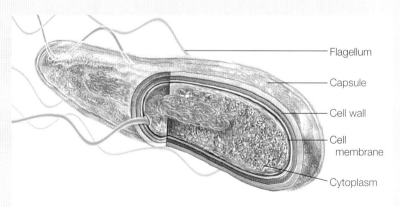

Our pal E. coli really furthers our cause when he brews up a nice batch of septicemia. We just love that guy!

A look at *Escherichia coli*

The most common cause of postoperative septicemia, *E. coli* is a common gram-negative bacilli that normally inhabits the GI tract. It's a simple rod-shaped one-celled microorganism with a cell wall that protects it from many of the human body's defense mechanisms. Although it doesn't have a nucleus, it does contain cytoplasm and possesses all the other mechanisms needed to survive and rapidly reproduce. The organism may be either nonmotile or motile, propelled by rotating flagella.

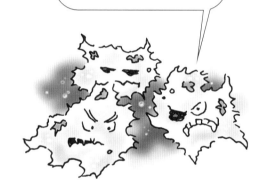

Flagellum

Capsule

Cell wall

Cell membrane

Cytoplasm

Septic shock

Septic shock occurs when bacteria release endotoxins into the bloodstream, decreasing vascular resistance and causing dramatic hypotension.

What to look for

Early signs and symptoms

- Fever
- Chills
- Warm, dry, flushed skin
- Slightly altered mental status
- Increased pulse and respiratory rates
- Decreased or normal blood pressure
- Reduced urine output

Late signs and symptoms

- Pale, moist, cold skin
- Deteriorating mental status
- Decreased pulse and respiratory rates
- Reduced blood pressure
- Decreased urine output

What to do

- Provide supplemental oxygen and prepare for ET intubation and mechanical ventilation.
- Administer I.V. antibiotics.
- Monitor vital signs and LOC.
- Monitor serum peak and trough levels.
- Give I.V. fluids and blood or blood products to restore circulating blood volume. If blood pressure remains low even after I.V. fluids and blood products have been administered, administer vasopressors.

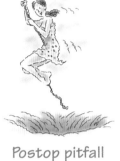

Postop pitfall

Understanding septic shock

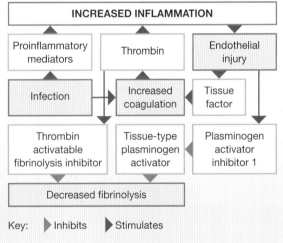

INCREASED INFLAMMATION		
Proinflammatory mediators	Thrombin	Endothelial injury
Infection	Increased coagulation	Tissue factor
Thrombin activatable fibrinolysis inhibitor	Tissue-type plasminogen activator	Plasminogen activator inhibitor 1
Decreased fibrinolysis		

Key: ▶ Inhibits ▶ Stimulates

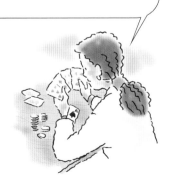

Don't gamble with septic shock. Provide supplemental oxygen; administer I.V. antibiotics; and monitor your patient's vital signs, LOC, and serum levels.

Thrombophlebitis

Postoperative venous stasis associated with immobility may lead to thrombophlebitis (inflammation of a vein, usually in the leg), possibly accompanied by clot formation.

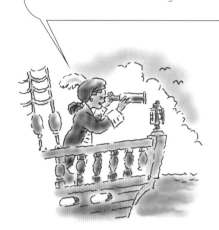

Inspect the patient's leg from foot to groin, and measure calf circumference. Note engorgement of the cavity behind the medial malleolus and increased temperature of the limb. Also check for cordlike venous segments.

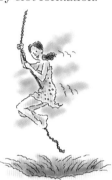

Postop pitfall
Assessing for thrombophlebitis

Thrombophlebitis may cause pain and tenderness in the calf, especially on dorsiflexion of the foot (Homan's sign).

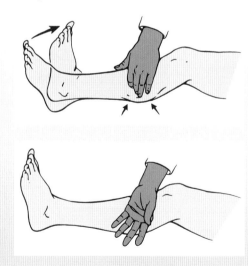

The affected limb may be warm to touch.

What to look for

■ Redness, swelling, and edema of the affected limb
■ Tenderness of the affected limb and a positive Homan's sign (pain on dorsiflexing the foot).
Note: These findings aren't always present.

What to do

■ Elevate the affected leg, and apply warm compresses.
■ Administer anticoagulants (initially heparin and, later, warfarin).
■ Monitor daily laboratory values, such as partial thromboplastin and prothrombin times and International Normalized Ratio.
■ If indicated, prepare the patient for surgical intervention with a vena cava filter to trap emboli and prevent pulmonary emboli.
■ After an acute episode, apply antiembolism stockings, and encourage ambulation.

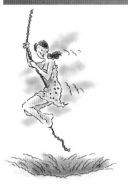

Postop pitfall
Venous thrombus

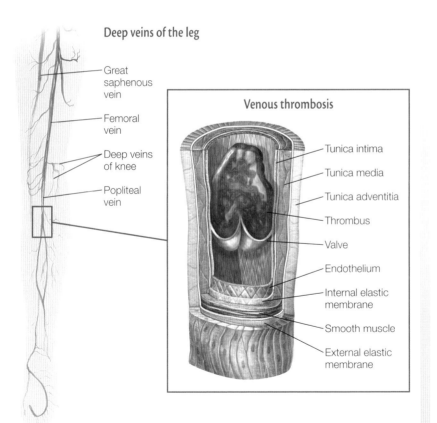

Deep veins of the leg

- Great saphenous vein
- Femoral vein
- Deep veins of knee
- Popliteal vein

Venous thrombosis

- Tunica intima
- Tunica media
- Tunica adventitia
- Thrombus
- Valve
- Endothelium
- Internal elastic membrane
- Smooth muscle
- External elastic membrane

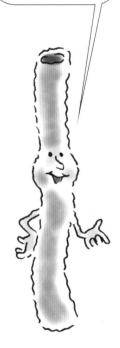

Watch out! There's a thrombus among us! Elevate the affected leg and give your patient anticoagulants.

Urine retention

For the first 12 hours after surgery, the patient may be unable to void spontaneously. However, urine retention is usually transient and reversible.

What to look for

- Absence of voiding
- Bladder distention above the symphysis pubis
- Complaints of discomfort and pain in the bladder area
- Anxiety and restlessness
- Diaphoresis
- Hypertension

What to do

- Help the patient ambulate as soon as possible after surgery (unless contra-indicated).
- Help the patient to a normal voiding position and then leave him alone (if possible) to void in private.
- If the patient still can't void despite these interventions, prepare for urinary catheterization.

Here are some tricks that might help your patient void: Turn on the water loud enough for her to hear, and pour warm water over the perineum.

Palpating the bladder

In a patient with urine retention, you may palpate a distended bladder in the abdominal area shown here.

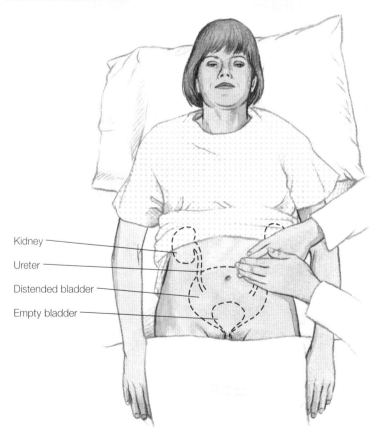

Kidney

Ureter

Distended bladder

Empty bladder

Wound dehiscence and evisceration

Occasionally, wound edges fail to join, or they separate even after they seem to be healing normally. Called *wound dehiscence*, this condition may lead to evisceration — a more serious complication in which a portion of the viscera protrudes through the incision. Evisceration, in turn, can result in peritonitis and septic shock.

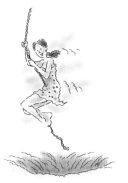

Using sterile technique, cover the extruding wound contents with warm sterile saline soaks.

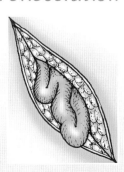

What to look for

■ Serosanguineous wound exudate (indicating dehiscence)
■ Visible coils of intestine (indicating evisceration)
■ Popping sensation felt by the patient after retching or forceful vomiting, coughing, or straining

What to do

■ Keep the patient in bed and stay with him while a colleague notifies the surgeon.
■ Withhold food and oral fluids in case the patient needs to return to the operating room.
■ Administer I.V. fluids to replace fluid lost from the wound.
■ Administer analgesics.

Postop pitfall

Recognizing wound dehiscence and evisceration

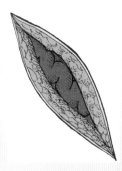

Wound dehiscence   Evisceration of bowel loop

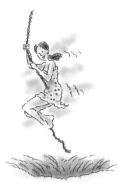

Postop pitfall
Wound dehiscence

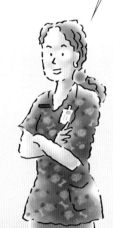

Wound dehiscence is a serious complication. Stay with the patient and have a colleague notify the surgeon.

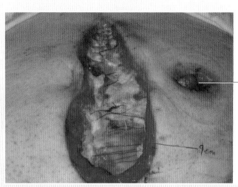

— Colostomy

Dehisced abdominal wound (with a colostomy)

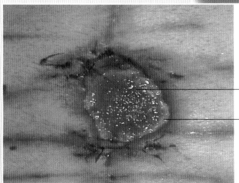

— Red granulation tissue

— Yellow fibrin slough

Dehisced healing abdominal incision

Wound infection

Wound infection is the most common type of wound complication. It's also a major factor in wound dehiscence and evisceration.

What to look for

■ Redness, increased tenderness, deep pain, edema, or discharge at the wound site
■ Increased pulse rate and temperature
■ Elevated white blood cell count

What to do

■ Obtain a wound specimen for culture and sensitivity testing.
■ Administer antibiotics.
■ Irrigate the wound with an appropriate solution.
■ Monitor wound drainage.

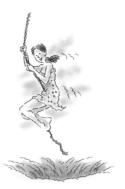

Postop pitfall

Early signs of wound infection

Watch for early signs of infection, such as redness and edema, at the wound site.

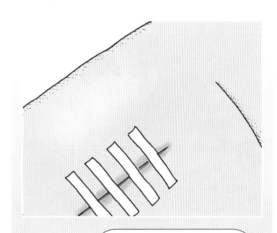

When assessing wound drainage, focus on color and consistency. Use the terms shown here as descriptors.

Wound drainage descriptors

Description	Color and consistency
Serous	■ Clear or light yellow ■ Thin and watery
Sanguineous	■ Red (with fresh blood) ■ Thin
Serosanguineous	■ Pink to light red ■ Thin and watery
Purulent	■ Creamy yellow, green, white, or tan ■ Thick and opaque

Patient discharge needs

JCAHO mandates that discharge planning begin early in the patient's stay. Optimally, you should have started planning for the patient's discharge at your first contact with him. Use your initial nursing history and preoperative assessment as well as subsequent assessments to determine your patient's readiness for discharge and what his needs will be once discharge is complete.

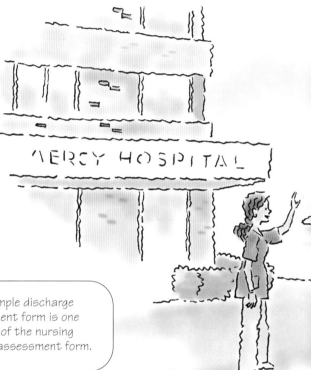

This sample discharge assessment form is one section of the nursing admission assessment form.

Discharge assessment questions

Discharge planning needs

Living arrangements (caregiver): _Sara Smith (patient's daughter)_

Type of dwelling: Apartment ☐ House ☑ Nursing home ☐ Boarding home ☐ Other _____

Physical barriers in home: No ☐ Yes ☑ Explain: _12-step flight of stairs to bathroom and bedroom_

Access to follow-up medical care: Yes ☑ No ☐ Explain: _____

Ability to carry out activities of daily living: Self-care ☐ Partial assistance ☐ Total assistance ☑

Needs help with: Bathing ☑ Eating ☑ Ambulation ☑ Other _____

Anticipated discharge destination: Home ☐ Rehab ☐ Nursing home ☑ Skilled nursing facility ☐ Boarding home ☐
Other _____

Preparing for the patient's homecoming

A home can be dangerous or inconvenient for someone recovering from surgery. Use this list to pinpoint household areas that the patient and his caregivers may need to adapt to fit his needs.

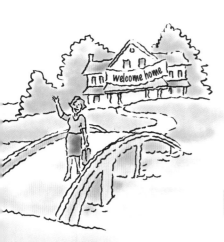

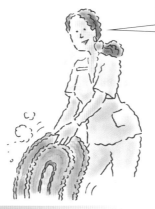

Kitchen

- Provide a working fire extinguisher.
- Reorganize storage areas.
- Install easy-to-reach stove controls.

All areas

- Install smoke and carbon monoxide detectors.
- Cover exposed heating pipes and radiators to prevent burns.
- Keep the indoor temperature no higher than 80° F (26.7° C) for maximum comfort.
- Provide good lighting.
- Install handrails along walls for support while walking.
- Provide low-pile carpeting for easy movement.
- Remove area and throw rugs, and keep floors clutter-free.
- Tape down loose carpet edges to prevent accidental trips and falls.
- Repair holes and rough floor areas.
- Install ramps over raised doorsills.
- Secure stair banisters and railings.
- Brightly tape step edges.
- Widen door frames to at least 27″ (68.6 cm) to accommodate a wheelchair.
- Provide a ramp leading into the house, and repair uneven spots on the steps and sidewalk.

Bedroom

- Keep a commode chair, urinal, or bedpan close to the bed.
- Provide a hospital-type bed (with side rails and attached trapeze).
- Install a bedside telephone.
- Provide a night-light or a bedside flashlight.
- Install a fire escape or portable ladder.

Living room

- Provide cushions to raise the seating level if the patient has trouble rising from a low chair or sofa.
- Arrange furniture to permit free access.
- Remove electrical cords and wires from walkways.
- Provide a conveniently located telephone (either stationary or portable) with a secured long cord (perhaps on a desk or table).

Bathroom

- Install grab bars in the shower and tub.
- Obtain a tub seat if the tub is difficult to enter and exit.
- Buy a shower chair for sitting instead of standing to bathe.
- Install a raised toilet seat.
- Put nonskid strips or a tub mat in the bathtub to prevent falls.
- Attach a handheld shower head for easy rinsing.
- Install easy-to-turn faucet handles.
- Hang mirrors, shelves, and racks at wheelchair level.
- Set the water heater temperature no higher than 120° F (48.9° C) to prevent burns.

Discharge summaries

Discharge summaries reflect the reassessment and evaluation components of the nursing process. JCAHO requires caregivers to document their assessment of the patient's continuing care needs and any referrals.

Many facilities combine discharge summaries and patient instructions in one form. This combined form has sections for recording patient assessment, patient teaching, detailed special instructions, and discharge circumstances. Make sure the completed form describes the patient's care, provides useful information for follow-up teaching and evaluation, and states that the patient has the information he needs to care for himself or get further help. Give one copy to the patient, and place another copy in his medical record.

Combined discharge summary and patient instructions

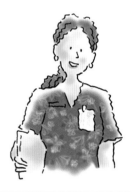

Discharge instructions

1. Summary Tara Nicholas is a 55-year-old woman with a history of hypertension admitted wih lung CA for ® lower lobectomy.
    Treatment: ® lower lobectomy
    Recommendation: Follow low-Na, low-cholesterol diet

2. Allergies penicillin

3. Medications (drug, dose time) Lopressor 25 mg by mouth at 6 am and 6 pm; temazepam 15 mg by mouth at 10 pm; Percocet 1 tab by mouth every 4 hours as needed for pain

4. Diet Low sodium, low cholesterol

5. Activity As tolerated

6. Discharged to Home

7. If questions arise, contact Dr. Pritchett Telephone number 555-1448

8. Special instructions Call MD for fever, ↑ tenderness, deep pain or drainage from incision site, or difficulty breathing.

9. Return visit Dr. Pritchett Place Surgical Care Clinic
    On date 3/15/06 Time 8:45 am

Tara Nicholas   JE Pritchett, MD

Signature of patient for receipt of   Signature of provider
   instructions from provider   giving instructions

> Have the patient or a family member read the medication instruction back to you.

> Write instructions clearly so the patient or family can easily understand them. This is the form they'll refer to when trying to remember your teaching.

Narrative discharge notes

If your facility uses narrative discharge notes instead of a combined form, make sure the completed notes include:
- patient status at time of admission and discharge
- significant information about the patient's stay, including resolved and unresolved patient problems and referrals for continuing care
- instructions given to the patient, family, or other caregivers about medications, treatments, activity, diet, referrals, follow-up appointments, and other special instructions.

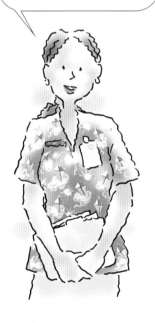

Some health care facilities use a narrative-style discharge summary, which is similar to a progress note. Here's a sample.

Narrative discharge notes

Date	Time	Progress notes
3/9/06	Discharge 1530 (summary)	41 y.o. black male admitted 3/3/06 with chest pain, hypertension; BP 190/100, and SOB. Emergent cardiac cath performed and pt. transported directly to OR for CABG. Pt. stable postop. Has been out of bed ambulating in the hallway. Incision clean and dry, without signs of infection. Reviewed drug regimen with pt. and wife. Both verbalized understanding of medication times, dosages, and adverse effects. Reviewed incision care and instructed pt. to notify MD of chest pain, SOB, fever, deep incisional pain or incisional drainage. Will call Dr. T. Harris for 5 day postdischarge appointment. Discharge instruction sheet given. ————————————— B. McCort, RN

VISION QUEST

Color my world

In this illustration of heart sound auscultation sites, color the aortic site blue, the pulmonic site green, the mitral site yellow, and the tricuspid site orange.

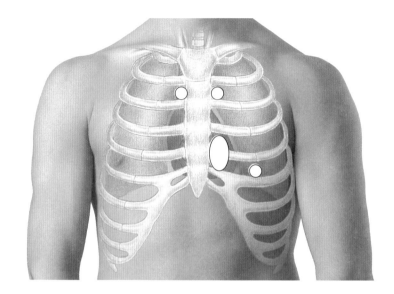

Matchmaker

Match the wound drainage descriptors on the left with their corresponding definitions.

1. Sanguineous

2. Purulent

3. Serous

4. Serosanguineous

A. Creamy yellow, green, white, or tan; thick and opaque

B. Red; thin

C. Pink to light red; thin, watery

D. Clear or light yellow; thin and watery

194

Selected references

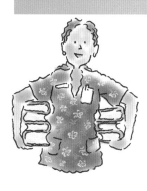

Alcenius, M. "Successfully Meet Pain Assessment Standards," *Nursing Management* 35(3):12, March 2004.

Barash, P.G., et al. *Handbook of Clinical Anesthesia*, 5th ed. Philadelphia: Lippincott Williams & Wilkins, 2006.

Blackbourne, L.H. *Advanced Surgical Recall*, 2nd ed. Philadelphia: Lippincott Williams & Wilkins, 2004.

DeFazio Quinn, D.M., and Schick, L. *PeriAnesthesia Nursing Core Curriculum: Preoperative, Phase I and Phase II PACU Nursing.* Philadelphia: W.B. Saunders Co., 2004.

Diehl-Oplinger, L., and Kaminski, M.F. "Choosing the Right Fluid to Counter Hypovolemic Shock," *Nursing2004* 34(3):52-54, March 2004.

Diseases, 4th ed. Philadelphia: Lippincott Williams & Wilkins, 2006.

Drain, C.B. *Perianesthesia Nursing: A Critical Care Approach*, 4th ed. Philadelphia: W.B. Saunders Co., 2003.

Dunn, D. "Preventing Perioperative Complications in Special Populations," *Nursing2005* 35(11):36-43, November 2005.

ECG Facts Made Incredibly Quick. Philadelphia: Lippincott Williams & Wilkins, 2006.

Ezekiel, M.R. *Handbook of Anesthesiology*, 2004-2005 ed. Laguna Hills, Calif.: Current Clinical Strategies Publishing, 2003.

Health Assessment Made Incredibly Visual. Philadelphia: Lippincott Williams & Wilkins, 2007.

Hohler, S. "Looking Into Minimally Invasive Total Hip Arthroplasty," *Nursing2005* 35(6):54-57, June 2005.

Hyett, J.M. "Caring for a Patient After CABG Surgery," *Nursing2004* 34(7):48-49, July 2004.

ISMP Medication Safety Alert! "Positive Identification: Not Just For Patients, But for Drugs and Solutions," *Nurse Advise-ERR* 3(8), August 2005.

Lawrence, P.F. *Essentials of General Surgery*, 4th ed. Philadelphia: Lippincott Williams & Wilkins, 2006.

Morton, P.G., et al. *Critical Care Nursing: A Holistic Approach*, 8th ed. Philadelphia: Lippincott Williams & Wilkins, 2005.

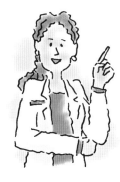

Muhlberg, A.H., and Ruth-Sahd, L. "Holistic Care Treatment and Interventions for Hypovolemic Shock Secondary to Hemorrhage," *Dimensions of Critical Care Nursing* 23(2):55-59, March-April 2004.

Mulholland, M.W., and Doherty, G.M. *Complications in Surgery.* Philadelphia: Lippincott Williams & Wilkins, 2006.

Mulholland, M.W., et al., eds. *Greenfield's Surgery: Scientific Principles & Practice,* 4th ed. Philadelphia: Lippincott Williams & Wilkins, 2006.

Nursing2007 Drug Handbook, 27th ed. Philadelphia: Lippincott Williams & Wilkins, 2007.

Pathophysiology: An Incredibly Easy Pocket Guide. Philadelphia: Lippincott Williams & Wilkins, 2006.

Potter, P.A., and Perry, A.G. *Fundamentals of Nursing,* 6th ed. St. Louis: Mosby–Year Book, Inc., 2005.

Rhoads, J. *Advanced Health Assessment and Diagnostic Reasoning.* Philadelphia: Lippincott Williams & Wilkins, 2006.

Rothrock, J.C. *Alexander's Care of the Patient in Surgery,* 12th ed. St. Louis: Mosby–Year Book, Inc., 2003.

Seal, L.A., and Paul-Cheadle, D. "A Systems Approach to Preoperative Surgical Patient Skin Preparation," *American Journal of Infection Control* 32(2):57-62, April 2004.

Smeltzer, S.C., and Bare, B.G. *Brunner & Suddarth's Textbook of Medical-Surgical Nursing,* 10th ed. Philadelphia: Lippincott Williams & Wilkins, 2004.

Ueda, K., et al. "A Comparative Study of Sequential Epidural Bolus Technique and Continuous Epidural Infusion," *Anesthesiology* 103(1):126-29, July 2005.

Credits

Chapter 1

"The Gross Clinic" (Thomas Eakins), page 2. Corbis.

Allis' ether inhaler, page 2. Courtesy of the National Library of Medicine.

U.S. Army General Hospital, 132nd, page 3. Courtesy of the National Library of Medicine.

Mallampati Airway Classification System, page 12. From Blackbourne, L.H., ed. *Advanced Surgical Recall*, 2nd ed. Philadelphia: Lippincott Williams & Wilkins, 2003.

Chapter 2

Stages of anesthesia, pages 22 and 23. Adapted with permission from Gillespie, N.A. "Signs of Anesthesia," *Anesthesia Analog* 22:275. © 1943.

Constant current nerve locator for regional blocks (Tracer® III Model NL-3), page 35. Life-tech, Inc.

Chapter 3

BD E-Z Scrub preoperative surgical scrub brushes, page 48. Courtesy and © Becton, Dickinson and Company.

Common surgical instruments, page 53. From Cohen, B.J. *Medical Terminology: An Illustrated Guide*, 4th ed. Philadelphia: Lippincott Williams & Wilkins, 2003.

Perioperative flow sheet, page 56. Adapted from the Association of Perioperative Registered Nurses' "Sample Intraoperative Patient Record."

Surgical skin preparation, page 59. From Blackbourne, L.H., ed. *Advanced Surgical Recall*, 2nd ed. Philadelphia: Lippincott Williams & Wilkins, 2003.

Chapter 4

Surgeon's view during arthroscopy, page 68. Courtesy of West Coast Radiology Center, Santa Ana, Calif.

Surgeon's view during rotator cuff repair, page 69. From Koval, K.J., and Zuckerman, J.D. *Atlas of Orthopaedic Surgery: A Multimedia Reference*. Philadelphia: Lippincott Williams & Wilkins, 2004.

MIDCAB procedure, page 87. Courtesy of Tufts-New England Medical Center.

Removing the recipient's heart, page 94. Becky Sell for *The Post* (an independent student-run newspaper serving Ohio University).

Picturing prosthetic valves, pages 120 and 121:

> Medtronic Hall prosthesis. © Medtronic. Used with permission.
>
> St. Jude Medical Regent Valve. © St. Jude Medical, Inc. 2006. This image is provided courtesy of St. Jude Medical, Inc. All rights reserved.
>
> Carpentier-Edwards Duraflex Low-Pressure Bioprosthesis Valve. Edwards Lifesciences, Irvine, Calif.
>
> Hancock II Bioprosthesis. © Medtronic. Used with permission.
>
> Carpentier-Edwards PERIMOUNT Pericardial Bioprosthesis Valve. Edwards Lifesciences, Irvine, Calif.

Chapter 5

Wong-Baker FACES pain rating scale, page 128. From Hockenberry, M.J., et al. *Wong's Essentials of Pediatric Nursing*, 7th ed. St. Louis: Mosby–Year Book, Inc., 2005. Used with permission. © Mosby.

We gratefully acknowledge Anatomical Chart Company and LifeART for the use of selected images.

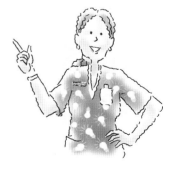

Index

A

Abdominal aortic aneurysm repair, 64-65
Abdominal quadrants, 154
Abdominal sounds, abnormal, 175
Abdominoperineal resection, 73
Abducens nerve, 152
acebutolol, 141
Acoustic nerve, 152
adenosine, 142
Adhesive skin closures, 159
Airway, evaluating, 12
alfentanil (Alfenta), 30
Altered arousal, stages of, 151
Ambulation, postoperative, 165
Ambulatory surgery, 3
American Nurses Association, 3
American Society of Anesthesiologists'
     Physical Status Classification, 13
Amidate, 27
Amides, 37
amiodarone, 142
Anacrotic limb, 129
Analgesia, 166, 167
Anastomosis, 72
Anectine, 33
Anesthesia, 2. See also specific type.
   balanced, 23
   basics of, 20
   levels of, 24
   types of, 21
Anesthesia complications, 135-144
Anesthesia evaluation, 12-13
Anesthetics, 25-37
Aneurysm
   abdominal aortic, repair of, 64-65
   cerebral, repair of, 82-83
Antiarrhythmic drugs, 141-142
Anticholinergic drugs, 34
Anticholinesterase drugs, 34
Appendectomy, 66-67
Arousal, altered, stages of, 151
Arrhythmias, postanesthesia, 137-140,
     141-142
Arterial pressure monitoring, 129
Arthroplasty, 102-103
Arthroscopy, 68-69
Asepsis, 3, 46-52
   draping and, 52
   gloving and, 50, 51
   gowning and, 48
   principles of, 46, 62
   scrubbing and, 47-48
Assessment
   discharge, 190
   postoperative, 125-134, 148-160
   preoperative, 8-11

Atelectasis, 168
atenolol, 141
atracurium (Tracrium), 33
Atrial fibrillation, postanesthesia, 139
Atrial flutter, postanesthesia, 139, 144
Atrial tachycardia, postanesthesia, 138
Atrioventricular block, postanesthesia,
     140, 146
atropine, 34, 35, 95, 142
Auscultation
   for breath sounds, 148-149
   for heart sounds, 150, 194

B

Bacteria, and postoperative infection,
     43, 62
Bag-valve mask device, 135
Barbiturates, 26
Bariatric surgery, 70-71
Bathroom, safety measures for, 191
Bedroom, safety measures for, 191
Benzodiazepine reversal agents, 31
Benzodiazepines, 28, 29
Bileaflet valve, 120
Biliopancreatic diversion, 71
Billroth operation, 92
Biopsy, breast tissue, 76
Bladder, palpating, 186
Blanket, postoperative, 143
Block, spinal, assessing level of, 134
Bovine valves, 121
Bowel resection, 72-75
Bowel sounds, abnormal, 175
Bradycardia, postanesthesia, 138
Breast cancer surgery, 76-77
Breath sounds, 148-149, 150
Brevital, 26
Bronchopneumonia, 169
Bruits, systolic, 175
bupivacaine, 36, 37
Burr holes, 88
Butterfly closures, 159
Bypass grafting
   coronary artery, 86-87
   femoral, 90-91

C

Carbocaine, 37
Carbolic acid, 3
Cardiac conduction system, 137
Cardiac output, 132
Cardiopulmonary bypass, 86
Cardiovascular system
   anesthesia complications and, 136-142
   preoperative assessment of, 10
   postoperative assessment of, 125, 150
Carotid endarterectomy, 78-79

Carpentier-Edwards Bioprosthesis
     valves, 121
Cataracts, 80-81
Catgut, 158
Catheter, pulmonary artery, 130, 144
Central venous pressure, 132
Cerebral aneurysm repair, 82-83
Chest auscultation, 148-149
Children, assessing pain in, 128
chloroprocaine (Nesacaine), 36, 37
Cholecystectomy, 84-85
Circle of Willis, 82
Circulating nurse, 3, 4
cisatracurium (Nimbex), 33
Cleanup, postoperative, 61
Closed-wound drainage system, 159
Colectomy, 72, 73
Colostomy formation, 74-75
Coma, 151
Commissurotomy, 118
Communication system, in operating
     room, 42
Compartment syndrome, 170-171
Confusion, 151
Coronary artery bypass grafting, 86-87
Coughing, 162
Crackles, 150
Cranial nerves, 152
Craniotomy, 88-89
Curare, 33
Cyanosis, 155

D

Decerebrate posture, 127
Decorticate posture, 127
Deep breathing, 162
Dehiscence, 187-188
Diagnostic testing, 7
diazepam (Valium), 28
Dicrotic limb, 129
Dicrotic notch, 129
diltiazem, 142
Diprivan, 27
Discharge
   from postanesthesia care unit, 145
   postoperative, 190-191, 192-193
Discharge planning, 15
Discharge summaries, 192-193
disopyramide, 141
Disorientation, 151
Dissociative agents, 27
Documentation
   discharge, 193
   of intake and output, 164
   perioperative, 60
   of pulses, 126
dofetilide, 142

doxacurium (Nuromax), 33
Drainage, wound, 187, 194
Drainage system, closed-wound, 159
Draping, 52, 59

E

Ears, preoperative assessment of, 10
Edema, 155
edrophonium (Tensilon, Enlon), 34
Electrical safety, in operating room, 42
Electrothrombosis, 83
Embolism. *See specific type.*
End diastole, 129
Endarterectomy, 78-79
Endoscopy, 3
Endotracheal intubation, 12
Endovascular grafting, 65
Enlon, 34
Epidural analgesia, postoperative, 167
Epidural anesthesia, 36, 38
epinephrine, 142
Escherichia coli infection, 182
esmolol, 141
Esophagojejunostomy, 93
Esters, 37
Ether, 2
etomidate (Amidate), 27
Evisceration, 187
Exercise, postoperative, 165
Eyes, preoperative assessment of, 10

F

Facial nerve, 152
Fat embolism, 172-173
Femoral bypass grafting, 90-91
fentanyl (Sublimaze), 30
Fibrillation, postanesthesia, 139, 140
Fixation devices, internal, for hip fracture
    repair, 99
flecainide, 141
Flow sheet
    perioperative, 56
    postanesthesia care unit, 125, 126
Fluid balance, postoperative, 164
flumazenil (Romazicon), 31
Food allergy screening, 11
Friction rub, 175, 176

G

Gallbladder removal, 84-85
Gastric binding, 70
Gastric bypass, 71
Gastric surgery, 92-93
Gastroduodenostomy, 92
Gastrointestinal system
    preoperative assessment of, 10
    postoperative assessment of, 125, 154
Gastrojejunostomy, 92

Gastroplasty, 70
General anesthesia
    agents for, 25-35
    goals of, 21
    stages of, 21-22, 38
Genitourinary system
    preoperative assessment of, 10
    postoperative assessment of, 154
Glasgow Coma Scale, 127
Glossopharyngeal nerve, 152
Gloving, 50, 51
glycopyrrolate (Robinul), 34
Gowning, 49
Grafting
    bypass, 86-87, 90-91
    endovascular, 65
Graft occlusion, 91

H

Hair removal, 55
Halothane, 25
Hand asepsis, 3
Hand scrubbing, 47, 48
Hand washing, 2
Health history, 8, 9
Heart rate, atropine and, 35
Heart sounds, 150, 194
Heart transplantation, 94-95
Heart valves, 118
    prosthetic, 120, 121
    replacing, 119
Heart-lung machine, 86
Hemicolectomy, 72, 73
Hemodynamic monitoring, 129-132
Hepatojejunostomy, 108
Herbs, and anesthesia interactions, 13
Hernia repair, 96-97
Herniated disk, 106
Hip joint fracture repair, 98-99
Hip replacement, 103
Homecoming, preparing for, 191
Humidity control, in operating room, 42
Hypertension, postanesthesia, 137
Hyperthermia, malignant, postanesthesia,
    143, 144
Hypoglossal nerve, 152
Hypotension, postanesthesia, 136
Hypothermia, postanesthesia, 143
Hypoventilation, postanesthesia, 135
Hypovolemia, 174
Hypovolemic shock, 174
Hysterectomy, 100-101

I

ibutilide, 142
Identification, patient, 16, 17
Ileal conduit, 116, 122
Ileal reservoir, 116, 117

Immunosuppressant drugs, 105
Incentive spirometry, 162-163
Incision, splinting, 166
Indiana pouch, 116
Infants, assessing pain in, 128
Infection, chain of, 44
Infection control, 43-45
Informed consent, 5
Inhalation anesthetic agents, 25
Instructions, patient, 192
Instruments, common, 53
Intake and output record, 164
Integumentary system
    preoperative assessment of, 10
    postoperative assessment of, 125, 155
Internal fixation devices, for hip fracture
    repair, 99
Intracranial pressure monitoring, 133
Intraoperative phase, of surgery, 6

J

Jackson-Pratt bulb drain, 159
Joint changes, degenerative, 103
Joint replacement, 102-103

K

Ketalar, 27
ketamine (Ketalar), 27
Kidney transplantation, 104-105
Kitchen, safety measures for, 191
Knee arthroscopy, 68
Knee replacement, 102, 122
Kock pouch, 116, 117

L

Laboratory tests, preoperative, 7
Laminectomy, 106-107
Laparoscopic surgery, 3
Laryngospasm, postanesthesia, 136
Laser technology, 3
Latex allergy screening, 11
Leg strength, assessing, 153
Lethargy, 151
lidocaine, 36, 37, 141
Lister, Joseph, 3
Liver transplantation, 108-109
Living room, safety measures for, 191
Lobectomy, 112
Local anesthesia, agents for, 37
Long, Crawford Williamson, 2
Lumpectomy, 76
Lung resection, 112-113

M

Malignant hyperthermia, postanesthesia,
    143, 144
Mallampati airway classification
    system, 12

Marcaine, 37
Mastectomy, 77
Mayo stand, 52, 53
Mean arterial pressure, 132
Medication safety, in operating room, 54
Medtronic Hall Prosthesis, 120
Medtronic Hancock II Valve, 121
mepivacaine (Carbocaine), 37
Mesh plug, for hernia repair, 97
methohexital (Brevital), 26
mexiletine, 141
Microdiskectomy, 106, 107
midazolam (Versed), 28
Miles' resection, 73
Minimally invasive direct coronary artery
    bypass, 86, 87
Minimally invasive surgery, 3
Mivacron, 33
mivacurium (Mivacron), 33
moricizine, 141
morphine, 30
Mucous fistula, 75
Muscle relaxants, 32-35
Muscle strength, grading, 126
Musculoskeletal injury, 153
Musculoskeletal system
    preoperative assessment of, 10
    postoperative assessment of, 125,
        126, 153

N

naloxone (Narcan), 31
Naropin, 37
Narrative notes, discharge, 193
Neonates, assessing pain in, 128
neostigmine (Prostigmin), 34
Neurologic system
    preoperative assessment of, 10
    postoperative assessment of, 125, 127,
        151-152
Neuromuscular blocker reversal agents,
    34-35
Neuromuscular blocking agents, 32-35
Nightingale, Florence, 3
Nimbex, 33
Norcuron, 33
Nose, preoperative assessment of, 10
Novocain
Numeric pain rating scale, 128
Nuromax, 33
Nursing diagnoses, 56
Nursing specialties, 3
Nutrition, postoperative, 164

O

Obtundation, 151
Oculomotor nerve, 152
Olfactory nerve, 152

Omniscience valve, 120
Operating room
    environmental factors in, 42
    patient arrival in, 56
    positioning patient in, 57
    setting up, 53-54
Operating room team, 4
Opioid agonists, patient teaching for, 166
Opioid reversal agents, 31
Opioids, 30
Optic nerve, 152
Organ rejection, preventing, 105
Ostomy, 74

P

Pain
    assessing, 160
    from herniated disk, 106
    incisional, 166
Pain management
    opioids and, 30
    postoperative, 166-167
Pain rating scales, 128
Pain transmission, 20
Pancreas-kidney transplantation, 104, 105
pancuronium, 33
Paralytic ileus, 175
Patient arrival, in surgical suite, 55-59
Patient instructions, discharge, 192
Patient teaching, preoperative, 14-15
Patient-controlled analgesia, 167
Pentothal, 26
Perianesthesia, basics of, 124
Pericardial friction rub, 176
Pericarditis, 176-177
Perioperative care, 39-62
    cleanup and, 61
    documenting, 60
    infection control and, 43-45
    operating room preparation and, 53-54
    patient arrival and, 55-59
    surgical asepsis and, 46-52
    surgical suite environment and, 40-42
Peripheral nerve stimulator, 35
Phacoemulsification, 80
Physical examination, preoperative, 10
Physical Status Classification, American
    Society of Anesthesiologists', 13
Pitting edema, 155
Pneumonectomy, 112, 113
Pneumonia, 168-169
Polyglycolic acid, 158
Pontocaine, 37
Porcine valves, 121
Positioning, patient, 57
Postanesthesia care unit
    arrival in, 124
    discharge criteria for, 145
    postoperative assessment in, 125-134

Postoperative care, 147-194
Postoperative phase, of surgery, 6
Postoperative team, 4
PQRST, for pain assessment, 160
Preference card, 53
Premature atrial contractions, post-
    anesthesia, 138
Premature ventricular contractions,
    postanesthesia, 139, 144
Preoperative care, 1-18
Preoperative phase, of surgery, 6
Preoperative team, 4
Pressure ulcers, 178-179
prilocaine (Citanest), 37
procainamide, 141
procaine, 36, 37
propafenone, 141
propofol (Diprivan), 27
propranolol, 141
Prostatectomy, 110-111
Prostigmin, 34
Pseudocholinesterase deficiency, 7
Pulmonary artery catheter, 130, 144
Pulmonary artery pressure, 132
Pulmonary artery waveforms, 131
Pulmonary artery wedge pressure, 131, 132
Pulmonary embolism, 180-181
Pulses, documenting, 126
pyridostigmine (Regonol), 34

Q

quinidine, 141

R

Range-of-motion exercises, 165
Reconstruction, breast, 77
Rectosigmoidostomy, 73
Regional anesthesia, agents for, 36
Regonol, 34
Renal system, postoperative assessment
    of, 125
Repositioning patient, 161
Reproductive system, preoperative
    assessment of, 10
Respiratory system
    anesthesia complications and, 135-136
    preoperative assessment of, 10
    postoperative assessment of, 125,
        148-150
Rhonchi, 150
Right atrial pressure, 132
Right ventricular pressure, 132
Risk factors, surgical, 8, 18
Robinul, 34
rocuronium (Zemuron), 33
Romazicon, 31
ropivacaine (Naropin), 37
Rotator cuff repair, 69

S

Safety measures, for homecoming, 191
Scrubbing, 47, 48
Scrub nurse, 3, 4
Sedation, levels of, 24
Semmelweis, Ignaz, 2
Septicemia, 182
Septic shock, 183
Shield mask, 47
Shoulder arthroscopy, 69
Shunt, in endarterectomy, 78
Sigmoid colon resection, 73
Sinus bradycardia, postanesthesia, 138
Sinus tachycardia, postanesthesia, 138
Skin closures, adhesive, 159
Skin preparation, 58
Skin turgor, assessing, 155
sotalol, 142
Spinal accessory nerve, 152
Spinal anesthesia, 36, 38, 134
Splinting, for incisional pain, 166
Sponge, herb-soaked, 2
Sterilizer, steam, 61
Steri-Strips, 159
St. Jude Medical Valve, 120
Stomas, intestinal, 74, 75, 116
Stroke volume, 132
Stupor, 151
Substance P, 30, 31
succinylcholine (Anectine), 32, 33
Sufenta, 30
sufentanil (Sufenta), 30
Surgery
    history of, 2-3
    phases of, 6
    risk factors for, 8
Surgical site, marking, 16
Surgical suite
    environmental factors in, 40-42
    patient arrival in, 56
Surgical team, 4
Sutures, 158
Systemic vascular resistance, 132
Systolic bruits, 175
Systolic peak, 129

T

Tachycardia, postanesthesia, 138, 139
Team, surgical, 4
Temperature control, in operating
    room, 42
Tensilon, 34
tetracaine, 36, 37
thiopental sodium (Pentothal), 26
Thoracoscopy, 113
Thoracotomy, 112-113
Throat, preoperative assessment of, 10

Thrombophlebitis, 184-185
Thyroidectomy, 114-115
Tilting-disk valve, 120
tocainide, 141
Tracrium, 33
Train-of-four stimulation, 35
Transcutaneous pacing, 95
Transplantation
    heart, 94-95
    kidney, 104-105
    liver, 108-109
Transurethral resection of prostate, 110
Trephine, 2
Trigeminal nerve, 152
Trochlear nerve, 152
tubocurarine (Curare), 33
Turning patient, 161

U

Urinary diversion, 116-117
Urine retention, 186

V

Vagus nerve, 152
Valium, 28
Valve repair, 118
Valve replacement, 119
Valvular surgery, 118-121
vasopressin, 142
vecuronium (Norcuron), 33
Venous hum, 175
Venous thrombus, 185
Ventilation system, in operating room, 42
Ventricular fibrillation, postanesthesia,
    140, 146
Ventricular tachycardia, post-
    anesthesia, 139
verapamil, 142
Verification, preoperative, 16-17
Versed, 28
Visual analog pain rating scale, 128

W

Warming blanket, 143
Waveforms, 129, 131, 133
Weight-loss surgery, 70-71
Wheezes, 150
Wong-Baker FACES pain rating scale, 128
Wound asepsis, 3
Wound assessment, 156-159
Wound dehiscence, 187-188
Wound drainage, 189, 194
Wound healing, 156, 157
Wounds, and postoperative infection,
    45, 189

XY

Xylocaine, 37

Z

Zemuron, 33

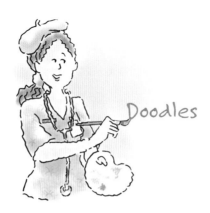

Doodles